CURRENT TOPICS IN GIARDIASIS

Edited by **Alfonso J. Rodriguez-Morales**

Current Topics in Giardiasis
http://dx.doi.org/10.5772/65182
Edited by Alfonso J. Rodriguez-Morales

Contributors

Amornnivit Kanokwanvimol, Joyce Siwila, Pablo Gortáres-Moroyoqui, Ana Balderrama-Carmona, Luis Leyva-Soto, Ruth Ulloa-Mercado, Edgar Morán-Palacio, Lourdes Mariana Díaz-Tenorio, Isaia Sotiriadou, Carmen Gallas-Lindemann, Poornima Sureshkumar, Michael J. Noack, Antonio Quispe, Wanderley De Souza, Marlene Benchimol, Víctor Molina, Alfonso J. Rodriguez-Morales

Published by InTech
Janeza Trdine 9, 51000 Rijeka, Croatia

Publishing Process Manager Maja Bozicevic
Technical Editor SPi Global
Cover InTech Design team

First published December, 2017
Printed in Croatia
Legal deposit, Croatia: National and University Library in Zagreb

Additional hard copies can be obtained from orders@intechopen.com

Current Topics in Giardiasis, Edited by Alfonso J. Rodriguez-Morales
p. cm.
Print ISBN 978-953-51-3653-8
Online ISBN 978-953-51-3654-5

For EU product safety concerns:
IN TECH d.o.o., Prolaz Marije Krucifikse Kozulić 3, 51000 Rijeka, Croatia,
info@intechopen.com or visit our website at intechopen.com.

Meet the editor

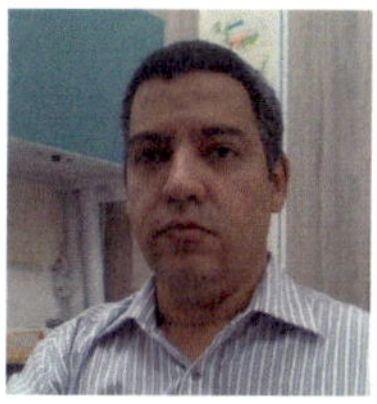

Prof. Alfonso J. Rodriguez-Morales received his Doctor of Medicine (MD) degree from the Universidad Central de Venezuela, Caracas, and he got his Master of Science (MSc) degree in Protozoology from the Universidad de Los Andes, Trujillo, Venezuela. He received his Diploma in Tropical Medicine and Hygiene (DTM&H) from the Universidad Peruana Cayetano Heredia, Lima, Peru, and University of Alabama at Birmingham, Birmingham, Alabama, USA. He is a fellow of the Royal Society for Tropical Medicine and Hygiene (FRSTMH), London, UK. He is a fellow of the Faculty of Travel Medicine (FFTM) of the Royal College of Physicians and Surgeons of Glasgow (RCPSG), Glasgow, Scotland, UK, and a fellow of the American College of Epidemiology (FACE), USA. Also, he is a Ph.D. candidate in Parasitology at the Universidad Central de Venezuela. Prof. Rodriguez-Morales is the president of the Travel Medicine Committee, Pan American ID Association. He is the secretary of the Colombian ID Association, a senior researcher of the Colciencias (2017–2019), and a professor in Universidad Tecnológica de Pereira, Pereira, Risaralda, Colombia (H index = 22).

Contents

Preface

Giardiasis is still a significant infectious and parasitic disease, caused by the protozoan *Giardia intestinalis* (syn. *G. duodenalis*, *G. lamblia*). Considered among the pathogens that probably were seen by Leeuwenhoek in 1681, the first descriptions were properly attributed to Vilèm Lambl in 1859. After centuries of advance in its knowledge, today we are aware that at least 8 different genotypes exist, ranging from A to H, being of human significance those included in A and B. However, other genotypes, in addition to other species in the genus, are significantly important in multiple other animal hosts. Among genotypes A and B, there are multiple subgenotypes that are important at the same time in other animals, e.g., dogs and cats, making giardiasis also a zoonotic disease. Although its historical importance, its epidemiology is not well understood, there is still a lack of national prevalence in multiple countries (1,2) and even more of molecular epidemiology identifying such genotypes. Despite that, there are estimates of more than 200 million of cases of giardiasis occurred in the world annually. Among those cases, although in tropical countries the prevalence tends to be higher, giardiasis is globally distributed. Recently its importance in new vulnerable populations has been recognized, which is the case, for example, of pregnant women (3) which are considered increasingly more exposed when visiting giardiasis-prevalent areas (4,5). Even more, in a globalized world, multiple infectious diseases have been linked to its occurrence to climate change and variability, also including giardiasis (5). Then, the advance in research in giardiasis during the last century and particularly during the last decade includes new forms of transmission (e.g., sexual transmission), as well the need for a world congress entirely dedicated to this pathogen (together with *Cryptosporidium*) (International Giardia & Cryptosporidium Conference, held now in seven occasions) (7).

At clinical level, giardiasis can lead to acute and chronic consequences, e.g., affecting children nutrition and development, as well as causing inflammatory intestinal syndrome and chronic fatigue, among multiple other sequelae (8-10). All these aspects call for the need of accurate and prompt diagnosis in order to provide effective treatments that can be prescribed as monotherapy of combination therapy (11,12).

With these conceptions in mind, this book includes different topics with regard to epidemiology, biology, clinical manifestations, treatment, and prevention, of the wide spectrum of manifestations caused by *Giardia* in humans and animals, trying to update the most significant research in many of them as well to offer a multinational perspective on different aspects. This book has been organized in three major sections: 1. "Overview, Epidemiology, and Clinical Aspects," 2. "Biological and Diagnostic Aspects," and 3. "Treatment, Prevention, and Public Health." Section I includes topics related to epidemiology and clinical aspects, including particularly the malabsorption syndrome and other aspects in livestock and companion animals. Section II includes basic aspects of *Giardia*, such as its cytoskeleton, the endomembrane system, and modern methods for its detection, such as the loop-mediate isothermal amplification. Finally, Section III discusses topics related to pharmacological management of this disease as well as the risk assessment in the environment.

Commissioning of this book by InTech editorial has been related in part to my long commitment with zoonotic parasitic and tropical diseases, being involved as the Co-Chair of the Working Group on Zoonoses of the International Society for Chemotherapy (WGZ-ISC), as well as in Colombia at the Committee on Zoonoses, Tropical Medicine and Travel Medicine of the Colombian Association of Infectious Diseases (Asociación Colombiana de Infectología, ACIN). Between 2009 and 2011, I was appointed as director of Population Studies and Epidemiology of national center for population studies in Venezuela (Fundacredesa), which performed the Second National Study of Human Growth and Development, including the survey for *Giardia* and other enteric parasites, which derived in multiple scientific analysis, products, and related publications on this and other protozoans and helminths.

After moving in 2011 to Colombia, I have been involved in research of parasitic diseases in Risaralda, where we still keep working on this important tropical disease. Part of all this is a clear reflect of the work impulse at the Research Group Infection Public Health and Infection of the Faculty of Health Sciences of the Universidad Tecnológica de Pereira, directed by Dr. Guillermo Javier Lagos-Grisales, not just a partner, a colleague, and mainly a friend but an extreme believer in our work in vector-borne and zoonotic diseases. But, I must recognize also the beginning of a significant collaboration after a meeting in Yokohama, Japan, during the International Congress of Chemotherapy, where I met Dr. Angel Arturo Escobedo, from Cuba, also part of the WGZ-ISC, who became since that year my most important collaborator on giardiasis. His work on giardiasis has kept me engaged also in this interesting parasitic disease.

Following the same philosophy as we had on my five previous books with InTech, *Current Topics in Tropical Medicine* (13), *Current Topics in Public Health* (14), *Current Topics in Echinococcosis* (15), *Current Topics in Chikungunya* (16), and *Current Topics in Malaria* (17), this book does not intend to be an exhaustive compilation, and this first edition has included not just multiple different topics but also a wide geographical participation from many countries of different regions of the world. Its on line availability through the website of InTech, as well the possibility to upload the complete book or their chapters in personal websites and institutions repositories, allows it to reach a wide audience in the globe. Continuing on the series of *Current Topics* books, we are planning to develop in the future other projects such as *Current Topics in Zika* (already in press, coming soon too), *Current Topics in Infectious Diseases*, and *Current Topics in Travel Medicine.*

I would like to give a very special thanks to InTechOpen (for the fourth time), and particularly to Maja Bozicevic and Romina Rovan (Publishing Process Managers), for the opportunity to edit this interesting and important book, as well for their constant support.

I want to take the appropriate time and space, as I used to do, to dedicate this book to my beloved family (Aurora, Alfonso José, Alejandro and Andrea, the neurologist) and particularly to my lovely wife, Diana. After 6 years together, I am so clear she is everything to me. She is the engine of my life. We have gone for difficult moments, partially related to my work, but our love has survived these challenges. And due to her support, projects like this one would be not just possible but successful. She is the highest blessing in my life, my soul mate and my strongest support for any journey; she provides everything in my life, day to day. Today, despite all that we have gone together, I cannot imagine my life without her. Also to my friends and my undergraduate and postgraduate students of health sciences in Colombia, Venezuela and around Latin America. Also it is time to say thanks to my colleagues at the Working Group on Zoonoses, International Society for Chemotherapy and the Committee on Zoonoses, Tropical Medicine and Travel Medicine (formerly on Zoonoses and Haemorrhagic Fevers) of the Colombian Infectious Diseases Society (ACIN). Special thanks are given to my friend and colleague Dr. Guillermo J. Lagos-Grisales, MD, MPH. Members of our research group and incubator consist of young and enthusiastic medical students and some veterinary medical students as well young medical doctors, who are pursuing significant improvements in the understanding of the epidemiology of zoonotic, vector-borne, parasitic and in general, infectious diseases, in our country with international projection. Year 2017 has been highly productive for this recognized group, which now is classified by the national agency of science, Colciencias, in the highest rank "A1," which is positioned as a leader in infectious disease epidemiology research in the coffee-triangle region and in the country.

Finally, I hope our readers enjoy this publication as much as I did reading the chapters of *Current Topics in Giardiasis*.

Prof. Alfonso J. Rodriguez-Morales
MD, MSc, DTM&H, FRSTMH (Lon), FFTM RCPS (Glasg), FACE, PhD (c)
Editor, Current Topics in Giardiasis
Part-Time Faculty Instructor, Risk Factors (Epidemiology) (Coordinator)
Department of Community Medicine, School of Medicine
Lecturer, Frontiers Research, School of Veterinary Medicine & Zootechnics
Director of Research, Faculty of Health Sciences, Universidad Tecnológica de Pereira
Pereira, Risaralda, Colombia
Co-Chair, Working Group on Zoonoses, International Society for Chemotherapy (ISC)
Secretary, Colombian Association of Infectious Diseases (ACIN)
Member of the Committee on Zoonoses, Tropical Medicine and Travel Medicine, ACIN
President, ACIN Chapter Coffee Triangle Region
President, Committee on Travel Medicine
Pan-American Association of Infectious Diseases
Senior Researcher, Colciencias (2017–2019)

References

[1] Rodríguez-Morales AJ, Granados-Álvarez S, Escudero-Quintero H, Vera-Polania F, Mondragon-Cardona A, Díaz-Quijano FA, Sosa-Valencia L, Lozada-Riascos CO, Escobedo AA, Liseth O, Haque U. Estimating and mapping the incidence of giardiasis in Colombia, 2009-2013. Int J Infect Dis. 2016 Aug;49:204-9.

[2] Quintero K, Durán C, Duri D, Medina F, Garcia J, Hidalgo G, Nakal S, Echeverria-Ortega M, Albano C, Incani RN, Cortez J, Jiménez S, Díaz M, Maldonado C, Matute F, Rodriguez-Morales AJ. Household social determinants of ascariasis and trichuriasis in North Central Venezuela. Int Health. 2012 Jun;4(2):103-10.

[3] Rodríguez-Morales AJ, Barbella RA, Case C, Arria M, Ravelo M, Perez H, Urdaneta O, Gervasio G, Rubio N, Maldonado A, Aguilera Y, Viloria A, Blanco JJ, Colina M, Hernández E, Araujo E, Cabaniel G, Benitez J, Rifakis P. Intestinal parasitic infections among pregnant women in Venezuela. Infect Dis Obstet Gynecol. 2006;2006:23125.

[4] Gallego V, Berberian G, Lloveras S, Verbanaz S, Chaves TS, Orduna T, Rodriguez-Morales AJ. The 2014 FIFA World Cup: communicable disease risks and advice for visitors to Brazil--a review from the Latin American Society for Travel Medicine (SLAMVI). Travel Med Infect Dis. 2014 May-Jun;12(3):208-18.

[5] Almanza C, Escobedo ÁA, Rodríguez-Morales AJ. Giardia infection in foreign visitors to Cuba. Travel Med Infect Dis. 2015 Nov-Dec;13(6):505-6.

[6] Escobedo AA, Almirall P, Rumbaut R, Rodríguez-Morales AJ. Potential impact of macroclimatic variability on the epidemiology of giardiasis in three provinces of Cuba, 2010-2012. J Infect Public Health. 2015 Jan-Feb;8(1):80-9.

[7] Escobedo AA, Arencibia R, Vega RL, Rodríguez-Morales AJ, Almirall P, Alfonso M. A bibliometric study of international scientific productivity in giardiasis covering the period 1971-2010. J Infect Dev Ctries. 2015 Jan 15;9(1):76-86.

[8] Durán C, Hidalgo G, Aguilera W, Rodriguez-Morales AJ, Albano C, Cortez J, Jiménez S, Díaz M, Incani RN. Giardia lamblia infection is associated with lower body mass in-dex values. J Infect Dev Ctries. 2010 Jun 30;4(6):417-8.

[9] Escobedo AA, Almirall P, Cimerman S, Rodríguez-Morales AJ. Sequelae of giardiasis: an emerging public health concern. Int J Infect Dis. 2016 Aug;49:202-3.

[10] Rodriguez-Morales AJ, Franco-Paredes C. Giardia Infections. In: Zhang Y (Editor). Encyclopedia of Global Health. ISBN 9781412941860. SAGE Publications, California, USA, 2008: Volume 2: 739. Available at: http://www.sage-ereference.com/abstract/globalhealth/n514.xml

[11] Escobedo AA, Lalle M, Hrastnik NI, Rodríguez-Morales AJ, Castro-Sánchez E, Cimerman S, Almirall P, Jones J. Combination therapy in the management of giardiasis: What laboratory and clinical studies tell us, so far. Acta Trop. 2016 Oct;162:196-205.

[12] Escobedo AA, Almirall P, Rodríguez-Morales AJ, Duquesne-Rivero E, Suarez-Mella R, Ruiz-Blanco E. Could the Fight Against Treatment Failures in Giardiasis Lead to a Second Childhood for Quinacrine? J Infect Dis. 2017 Aug 3. doi: 10.1093/infdis/jix375.

[13] Rodriguez-Morales AJ. (Editor). Current Topics in Tropical Medicine. ISBN 978-953-51-0274-8. InTech, Croatia, March 2012. Available at: http://www.intechopen.com/books/current-topics-in-tropical-medicine

[14] Rodriguez-Morales AJ. (Editor). Current Topics in Public Health. ISBN 978-953-51-1121-4. InTech, Croatia, May 2013. Available at: http://www.intechop-en.com/books/current-topics-in-public-health

[15] Rodriguez-Morales AJ. (Editor). Current Topics in Echinococcosis. ISBN 978-953-51-2159-6. InTech, Croatia, September 2015. http://www.intechopen.com/books/current-topics-in-echinococcosis

[16] Rodriguez-Morales AJ. (Editor). Current Topics in Chikungunya. ISBN 978-953-51-2595-2. InTech, Croatia, August 2016. http://www.intechopen.com/books/current-topics-in-chikungunya

[17] Rodriguez-Morales AJ. (Editor). Current Topics in Malaria. ISBN 978-953-51-2790-1. InTech, Croatia, November 2016. http://www.intechopen.com/books/current-topics-in-malaria

Section 1

Overview, Epidemiology and Clinical Aspects

Chapter 1

Introductory Chapter: Giardiasis - Still a Globally Relevant Protozoan and Zoonotic Disease

Alfonso J. Rodríguez-Morales, Adriana M. Trujillo,
Jorge A. Sánchez-Duque and Ángel A. Escobedo

Additional information is available at the end of the chapter

http://dx.doi.org/10.5772/intechopen.70900

1. Introduction

Giardiasis continues to be a significant parasitic disease in the world caused by the species of *Giardia* genus, particularly *Giardia intestinalis*, which affects humans and animals in a wide clinical spectrum, with zoonotic potential due to shared genotypes that can affect the same hosts. This protozoan disease occurs in developing as well as in industrialized countries, also affecting travelers. In recent years, multiple aspects in its epidemiology, but also and particularly in the long-term clinical consequences, have been highlighted. In this introductory chapter, a review on general aspects, based on recent experiences, is described.

2. Overview and general aspects of giardiasis

Giardia was described and was associated with the symptoms in 1681 for the first time when the Dutchman, Van Leeuwenhoek, found the trophozoites in his own feces; nevertheless, just until 1859, the first report was credited to the Czech Vilém Lambl [1–3]. *Giardia intestinal* is a flagellated protozoon (also known as *G. lamblia* or *G. duodenalis*) and is a tiny and ubiquitous intestinal and/or biliary parasite, which affects mammals, such as humans, pets, and livestock by inhabiting the upper part of the small intestine [4–6]. Frequently, this parasite contaminates water sources worldwide especially in temperate and tropical locations where sanitary conditions are suboptimal; for this reason, giardiasis is the commonest parasitic infection of the gastrointestinal tract, the most important responsible for outbreaks of diarrhea and sporadic endemic disease [7, 8].

3. Epidemiology

Distributed worldwide, *Giardia* is probably the most frequent pathogenic intestinal protozoon in children and adults, and one of the most common nonviral causes of diarrhea, afflicting annually an approximate 280 million individuals. Due to its intensifying global burden and its developmental and socioeconomic impact on infected individuals, this parasitosis was incorporated in the Neglected Disease Initiative of the World Health Organization in 2004 [4, 7, 9, 10].

In developed countries, giardiasis is associated with social and climatic factors and is referred as a re-emerging infectious agent. Some epidemiological studies have shown that its prevalence varies between the population studied and the location, from 2 to 5% on industrialized countries to 20–30% in developing countries [1, 5, 11], and these changes in prevalence are associated, among others, with the hygiene infrastructure and the impact of the weather conditions, reason why environmental control efforts are necessary, which requires an integrated and systematic approach to decrease and mitigate the influence on the disease epidemiology; for this reason, it is linked to educational programs and other interventional measures [2, 6, 12].

Although in Latin America, a restricted quantity of population-based studies has been performed, in Cuba, according to the last national intestinal parasites survey (n = 5850), the prevalence of *Giardia lamblia* infection was determined to be at 6.02% (95%CI 5.40–6.63) [13].

This parasitosis is highly infectious where *Giardia* cysts are habitually excreted in considerable population, especially in young children after ingestion of contaminated water or food and through person-to-person contact. Cysts can survive for months in cold water, and they are relatively resistant to chlorination, reason why between 10 and 100 cysts are sufficient to establish infection 100% of the time. Consequently, ingestion of water or food that contains small levels of contamination can result in the disease, which is more recurrent in summer and fall. Other usual ways to transmit them could be among day care center attendees and people who live in residential institutions, and it could also spread by means of sexual activity, by oral-anal contact [1, 5, 11, 12].

4. Life cycle

Giardia intestinalis is a noninvasive protozoan parasite with a simple life cycle and a simplified metabolism that depends on the host for nutrients such as purines, pyrimidines, cysteine, and cholesterol. The genus *Giardia* and its life cycle are relatively well recognized and clearly defined; members of the genus are flagellated protozoans belonging to the class Zoomastigophorea and order Diplomonadida, which lives and multiplies by asexual multiplication frequently on the luminal surface of the small intestine of its vertebrate host [14–16].

The trophozoite, which is 9–21 μm long, 5–15 μm wide, and 2–4 μm thick, lives in the small intestine and is responsible for many manifestations of the disease. The cytoskeleton composed of unique families of structural proteins and carbohydrates involves two nuclei, a ventral sucking adhesive disk by which it may adhere to intestinal epithelial cells, a median body, and four pairs of flagella that behave differently during motility. The dorsal surface is pear shaped and bilaterally symmetrical, with the two highly characteristic nuclei best visualized after staining. The newly emerged trophozoites infect the duodenum and jejunum where there is a favorable alkaline pH; they attach intimately to the intestinal epithelium by their ventral disk and begin to multiply by binary fission. Detection of soluble cyst wall proteins in the feces forms the basis of many stool antigen assays [1, 8, 16, 17].

Giardia takes advantage of host conditions at each step of its descent through the human gastrointestinal tract. After ingestion, *Giardia* infection is initiated by the acidic milieu in the stomach and the presence of bile and trypsin in the duodenum, and then, it reproduces in the small intestine, yielding two trophozoites from each cyst, which quickly divide again. Exposure of cysts to gastric acid triggers excystation, although the "excyzoites" do not emerge from the cyst until it passes into the small intestine. In vitro trophozoites double in number every 6 hours in the fastest growing isolates. The emerging parasites (excyzoites) quickly transform into trophozoites that attach to the intestinal epithelial cells using the adhesive disk, which is a major virulence factor; in this way, any excreted cysts are mature, highly infectious, and quite resistant to disinfectants routinely used for water treatment such as chlorine [8, 16, 18].

When the trophozoite senses a change in the environment as the cell is transported further down in the small intestine, it starts the encystation; in the earliest moment of this process, some specific vesicles are designed that allow its development and maturation, probably as a result of cholesterol starvation. At the same time with several proteins implicated in metabolic pathways, after that, several proteins also change their expression by important gene expression changes. *Giardia* has a considerable metabolic capacity as another parasite that lacks pathways for de novo biosynthesis of pyrimidines and purines for nucleotide salvage, but this process is conditioned by oxygen concentration, despite anaerobic metabolism and generating reactive oxygen species (ROS) by the host [1, 14–17].

Giardiasis as a multifactorial disease involves in its pathobiology complex interactions between host and parasite, differences in nutritional status, immune status, co-infections, and intestinal normal flora that could contribute to the differences in disease outcome observed among individuals from developing against developed countries. The roles of the host's intestinal normal flora and co-infections during *Giardia* infections are still largely unascertained [3, 12, 15, 19].

Some morphologically identical but genetically distinct *Giardia* infect humans and animals that now are divided into eight assemblages (A–H) what could bring a clarification about infection outcome. Thus, assemblages A and B are found in human and other animals, being considered zoonotic, whereas the other assemblages display host specificity and do not infect humans (C and B in dog, F in cat, E in hoofed animal, G in rodents, and H in sea mammals). Interestingly, this proportion is not altered when comparing data from developing and developed countries, but the prevalence of mixed infections is higher in the developing countries [8, 15–18].

The two assemblages (A and B) are composed of genetically distinguishable isolates, which may vary in infectivity, antigenicity, and virulence. In addition, human hosts vary in susceptibility to infection and disease and in the response to tolerance to infection. In this way, *Giardia* is an intraluminal parasite that adheres to the epithelium by way of an adhesive or sucking disk, although invasion of the epithelium either does not occur or is rare. Meanwhile, the number of trophozoites in the intestine can be so large that adherent organisms cover much of the epithelial surface. This could disrupt the epithelial brush border and contribute to lack of disaccharidase as could be seen in some patients [8, 14, 15].

5. Clinical aspects

The clinical manifestations, course, and duration of *Giardia* infections are variable. In that way, infections may be self-limited or persistent, asymptomatic, or symptomatic. Usually, most patients remain asymptomatic, but when signs and symptoms occur and acute disease is established, manifestations happen normally in travelers and in outbreaks, and they are characterized by diarrhea, nausea, anorexia, dehydration, flatulence, eructation, distention, abdominal cramping, and weight loss. Contradictorily, fever and vomiting are uncommon [7, 13, 20].

The first signs of infection appear after 6–15 days. Most symptomatic infections resolve spontaneously; however, sometimes, hospitalization is required when infections have long-term consequences and do not respond to the normal treatment. Chronic *Giardia* infections are reported frequently in nonendemic areas and also could result in irritable bowel syndrome, food allergies, arthritis, aphthous ulcers, or chronic fatigue syndrome after resolution [3, 10–12].

In some cases, if acute symptoms are not treated on time, they can develop into a chronic stage, which can affect all age groups but children are at higher risk, in whom *Giardia* infections have been associated with lower serum level of zinc, iron, and vitamins (A, B12, and folate); despite similar anthropometric indicators among infected and uninfected individuals in early childhood, the failure to thrive and poor cognitive function are characteristics in them. Furthermore, the loss of lactose is common and can persist for some weeks after treatment, which is why it is necessary to be distinguished in symptomatic patients from relapse or reinfection. In extreme cases, malabsorption and weight loss are severe and mimic sprue [1, 2, 8].

A typical scenario is a mildly to moderately ill person who grumbles of a raised number of urgent loose stools, with flatus, cramping, anorexia, and weight loss. There may even be periods when the person feels better only to relapse and then become noticeably worse. Finally, after some days to several weeks, the person will seek medical help. Similar to other causes of infectious diarrheas, symptoms can carry on after successful treatment and evolve into irritable bowel syndrome and chronic fatigue, even 6 years after the infection. Infrequently, *Giardia* is also found in biliary and pancreatic ducts and can cause cholecystitis and pancreatitis, and other localizations reported are the urinary tract, gastric mucosa, and colonic and ileal mucosa. Extraintestinal manifestations and long-term consequences are unusual, but a series of sporadic cases documented them in a third of the patients. The signs can include rash, reactive arthritis, eye complaints, and cognitive deficiencies [1, 2, 9, 10, 20].

6. Diagnostics

The diagnosis of giardiasis is based on the detection of cysts, trophozoites, or parasite-specific antigens in fecal microscopic examination, complemented with microscopic examination of duodenal fluids or in other biological samples. Polymerase chain reaction has been largely experimental, but it is being increasingly used in field and laboratory settings; considering that excretion of cysts may be variable or in low concentrations (50–80% sensitive), two or three checkups may be necessary, leading to a late diagnosis (>2 weeks) [3]. Stool antigen tests are standard in most laboratories and are highly sensitive (>90%), specific (~100%), and relatively inexpensive and do not require a trained microscopist [2, 9, 13, 18].

The observation of small intestine biopsy specimens or intestinal contents for trophozoites was the previous "gold standard" for diagnosis, but now, it is uncommonly needed to establish or to confirm the diagnosis. A number of morphological characteristics of the trophozoite can be used for the initial diagnostic, but it is not possible to identify which specific species by light microscopy, the reason why another type of test could be used in the medical approach. Electron microscopy might be useful for the identification of some *Giardia* species, but it is not applicable for screening or routine use [15, 18].

The use of immunological methods offers an important alternative for the diagnosis. The use of fluorescence microscopy and the direct fluorescence antibody test, which recognizes surface epitopes on cysts, has been reported to achieve relatively high specificity (99.8–100%) and sensitivity (93–100%) for the detection. The detection of *Giardia* antigens in fecal samples is another approach. Various enzyme-linked immunoassays have been used and report specificities of 87–100% and sensitivities of 63–100%. Flow cytometry is another technique to identify the *Giardia* cysts when immunofluorescent staining and microscopic examination and/or enumeration report unsatisfactory results [15, 18].

In some cases, the laboratory findings are nonspecific, and in low-intensity infections, testing methods can be false negative for which it is required to repeat the test. On the other hand, the white blood cell count and liver function test results used to be normal. The electrolyte disturbances could be present if diarrhea and vomiting are severe. White blood cells, lactoferrin, blood, and mucus are not found in stools. Immunoglobulin levels are usually normal but usually low or absent in susceptible hypogammaglobulinemic individuals [2, 3].

7. Treatment

During the last 60 years of the past century, the arsenal of antigiardial drugs has been increasing, and they still are in use. Before the introduction of quinacrine, these infections were treated with mercury, carbon tetrachloride, arsenicals, and bismuth; at present, an important number of agents have shown to be efficacious against *Giardia* in vitro and clinically. Nevertheless, current investigations try to establish an appropriate treatment regimen in giardiasis, but none of them appear to fulfill most of the criteria for an ideal drug. In fact, giardiasis is regularly considered an easily treated infection, but at times, due to treatment failure, re-infection or postinfection syndromes can have a huge impact on quality of life of the patient, which is why it is important to know at least six different classes of drugs, with different mechanisms, indication, and contraindications [1, 2, 21].

The 5-nitroimidazole (5-NI) derivatives remain the most frequently prescribed drugs, as well as metronidazole, tinidazole, and secnidazole. In spite of their efficacy, the treatment with these drugs is associated with several adverse effects, which are not always tolerable such as headache, metallic or bitter taste in mouth, nausea, vomiting, diarrhea, dizziness, general body discomfort, loss of appetite, etc. Whereas medical opposition may limit the use of some of them in singular cases, as in pediatrics, where their dose requirements make difficult the administration of tablet formulations to children. Finally, in the follow-up of some patients after treatment to evaluate the response to antigiardial drugs, a therapeutic failure is identified [4, 7, 21, 22].

Nitazoxanide is a new very broad spectrum 5-nitrothiazolyl derivative with a potentially useful activity against a range of biological agents. The effect of nitazoxanide in *Giardia* trophozoite includes ultrastructural changes in the cell morphology, swelling, and the formation of large empty areas in the cytoplasm and the disruption of the plasma membrane. An overall response rate of 75–94%, usually well tolerated, and a few adverse effects are the reason to choose this medicament [1, 22].

Some patients, who are being treated with the standard treatment that cures other patients, can continue with symptoms. In these cases, there are possibilities of different situations, including drug resistance, cure followed by reinfection, and also noncompliance and post-*Giardia* lactose intolerance, because when a drug-resistant giardiasis is identified, the stage changes and it is necessary to use another antigiardial compound with a different mechanism of action or a drug combination [1, 2, 4].

When there is a resistant *Giardia*, some therapeutic strategies could be used, since increasing the alternative dose and/or duration of the same one, changing another antigiardial, or using a drug combination might exert the synergistic effects. For this reason, the combination of the therapy should be reserved when single primary agents have failed to clear the infection. However, it also should be considered that administration of two or three drugs may have more profound physiological consequences, alter the intestinal microbiota, and increase the drug-related adverse events and health care costs [8, 9, 22].

8. Control and prevention

The interest in *Giardia* infection studies have been raising since its inclusion in the World Health Organization (WHO) in the Neglected Diseases Initiative in 2004 [9, 19]. In the same way, a bibliometric study of scientific production on giardiasis reports 6964 papers between 1971 and 2010 available in PubMed, written in 27 different languages corresponding to original articles (78.5%), reviews (8.6%), case reports (6.8%), and letters to the editors (3.6%) that evidenced a steady growth of literature dedicated to *Giardia* and its infection throughout the 40-year analyzed period [7].

This pathogen has been highlighted for the importance in terms of patient well-being and its effects on quality of life for being a continuing cause of the patient's discomfort and pain. Unfortunately, due to a lack of political will, funding, interest from the scientific community, or the combination of all of these factors, giardiasis is not a health priority; that is why, it is important to take in mind that this infection is prevented by a scrupulous personal hygiene, proper disposal of sewage, removal or killing of cysts from water supplies, and preventing contamination of food and water [2, 20].

Actually, the global burden of chronic giardiasis is not known, and the difficulties in diagnostic tools, the lack of definition, and difficulties to quantify the impact of an infection that causes an acute or chronic one, principally symptomatic illness, contribute to the necessity to realize studies that estimate the problems in terms of cost, day lost for disability, and quality of life [9, 18].

Despite that, important contributions have been made regarding the spectrum of illness attributable to giardiasis. It is illustrated in the protective effect of *Giardia* against other types of diarrhea what could be due to the anti-inflammatory activity of *Giardia*. Nevertheless, further investigations on the pathogenic mechanisms are needed that could lead to potential interventions preventing the severe illness [2, 11].

Author details

Alfonso J. Rodríguez-Morales[1,2,3,4]*, Adriana M. Trujillo[1], Jorge A. Sánchez-Duque[1] and Ángel A. Escobedo[3,4,5]

*Address all correspondence to: arodriguezm@utp.edu.co

1 Public Health and Infection Research Group, School of Medicine and School of Veterinary Medicine and Zootechnics, Faculty of Health Sciences, Universidad Tecnológica de Pereira, Pereira, Risaralda, Colombia

2 Committee on Zoonoses and Haemorrhagic Fevers, Asociación Colombiana de Infectología, Bogotá, DC, Colombia

3 Working Group on Zoonoses, International Society for Chemotherapy, Aberdeen, United Kingdom

4 Committee on Clinical Parasitology, Pan-American Association of Infectious Diseases, Panama City, Panama

5 Department of Parasitology, Academic Paediatric Hospital "Pedro Borrás," La Habana, Cuba

References

[1] Escobedo AA, Cimerman S. Giardiasis: A pharmacotherapy review. Expert Opinion on Pharmacotherapy. 2007;**8**(12):1885-1902

[2] Robertson LJ, Hanevik K, Escobedo AA, Morch K, Langeland N. Giardiasis—Why do the symptoms sometimes never stop? Trends in Parasitology. 2010;**26**(2):75-82

[3] Almirall P, Alfonso M, Ávila I, Salazar Y, Escobedo AA, Núñez FA, et al. Variaciones en las manifestaciones clínicas de la giardiosis en pacientes pediátricos hospitalizados, según grupos de edades. Revista Chilena de Infectología. 2013;**30**(5):502-506

[4] Pasupuleti V, Escobedo AA, Deshpande A, Thota P, Roman Y, Hernandez AV. Efficacy of 5-nitroimidazoles for the treatment of giardiasis: A systematic review of randomized controlled trials. PLoS Neglected Tropical Diseases. 2014;**8**(3):e2733

[5] Escobedo AA, Almirall P, Alfonso M, Cimerman S, Chacin-Bonilla L. Sexual transmission of giardiasis: A neglected route of spread? Acta Tropica. 2014;**132**:106-111

[6] Ryan U, Caccio SM. Zoonotic potential of *Giardia*. International Journal for Parasitology. 2013;**43**(12-13):943-956

[7] Escobedo AA, Arencibia R, Vega RL, Rodriguez-Morales AJ, Almirall P, Alfonso M. A bibliometric study of international scientific productivity in giardiasis covering the period 1971-2010. Journal of Infection in Developing Countries. 2015;**9**(1):76-86

[8] Escobedo AA, Lalle M, Hrastnik NI, Rodriguez-Morales AJ, Castro-Sanchez E, Cimerman S, et al. Combination therapy in the management of giardiasis: What laboratory and clinical studies tell us, so far. Acta Tropica. 2016;**162**:196-205

[9] Escobedo AA, Hanevik K, Almirall P, Cimerman S, Alfonso M. Management of chronic *Giardia* infection. Expert Review of Anti-infective Therapy. 2014;**12**(9):1143-1157

[10] Halliez MC, Buret AG. Extra-intestinal and long term consequences of *Giardia* duodenalis infections. World Journal of Gastroenterology. 2013;**19**(47):8974-8985

[11] Rodriguez-Morales AJ, Granados-Alvarez S, Escudero-Quintero H, Vera-Polania F, Mondragon-Cardona A, Diaz-Quijano FA, et al. Estimating and mapping the incidence of giardiasis in Colombia, 2009-2013. International Journal of Infectious Diseases: IJID: Official Publication of the International Society for Infectious Diseases. 2016;**49**:204-209

[12] Escobedo AA, Almirall P, Rumbaut R, Rodriguez-Morales AJ. Potential impact of macroclimatic variability on the epidemiology of giardiasis in three provinces of Cuba, 2010-2012. Journal of Infection and Public Health. 2015;**8**(1):80-89

[13] Almanza C, Escobedo AA, Rodriguez-Morales AJ. *Giardia* infection in foreign visitors to Cuba. Travel Medicine and Infectious Disease. 2015;**13**(6):505-506

[14] Thompson RC, Monis PT. Variation in *Giardia*: Implications for taxonomy and epidemiology. Advances in Parasitology. 2004;**58**:69-137

[15] Einarsson E, Ma'ayeh S, Svard SG. An up-date on *Giardia* and giardiasis. Current Opinion in Microbiology. 2016;**34**:47-52

[16] Birkeland SR, Preheim SP, Davids BJ, Cipriano MJ, Palm D, Reiner DS, et al. Transcriptome analyses of the *Giardia lamblia* life cycle. Molecular and Biochemical Parasitology. 2010;**174**(1):62-65

[17] Carranza PG, Lujan HD. New insights regarding the biology of *Giardia* lamblia. Microbes and Infection. 2010;**12**(1):71-80

[18] Koehler AV, Jex AR, Haydon SR, Stevens MA, Gasser RB. *Giardia*/giardiasis—A perspective on diagnostic and analytical tools. Biotechnology Advances. 2014;**32**(2):280-289

[19] Duran C, Hidalgo G, Aguilera W, Rodriguez-Morales AJ, Albano C, Cortez J, et al. *Giardia* lamblia infection is associated with lower body mass index values. Journal of infection in developing countries. 2010;**4**(6):417-418

[20] Escobedo AA, Almirall P, Cimerman S, Rodriguez-Morales AJ. Sequelae of giardiasis: An emerging public health concern. International Journal of Infectious Diseases: IJID: Official Publication of the International Society for Infectious Diseases. 2016;**49**:202-203

[21] Escobedo AA, Ballesteros J, Gonzalez-Fraile E, Almirall P. A meta-analysis of the efficacy of albendazole compared with tinidazole as treatments for *Giardia* infections in children. Acta Tropica. 2016;**153**:120-127

[22] Rodriguez-Morales AJ, Martinez-Pulgarin DF, Munoz-Urbano M, Gomez-Suta D, Sanchez-Duque JA, Machado-Alba JE. Bibliometric assessment of the global scientific production of nitazoxanide. Cureus. 2017;**9**(5):e1204

Chapter 2

Giardiasis Epidemiology

Antonio Marty Quispe Gutiérrez

Additional information is available at the end of the chapter

http://dx.doi.org/10.5772/intechopen.70338

Abstract

Giardiasis is the intestinal infection caused by *Giardia lamblia*, in which pathogenicity was cast doubted for decades but now is recognized as one of the most common causes of diarrheal disease worldwide. Originally described as waterborne transmitted, it has been broad described as of fecal-oral, person-to-person contact, and sexual transmission also. Although it is recognized as endemic throughout the world, most cases are reported from tropical countries with regular outbreaks commonly reported from developed countries. In humans, giardiasis normally produces a self-limited infection without symptoms, but some patients may present intestinal symptoms such as diarrhea and abdominal pain, and few show symptoms long after parasites clear up. Upon diagnosis, we may choose among several effective treatment alternatives, but not every patient responds to such therapies. Hence, having specific knowledge about the epidemiology of *Giardia*, it is critical for its prevention, which is the best strategy to protect us against such important disease.

Keywords: giardiasis, *Giardia*, *Giardia lamblia*, epidemiology, life cycle stages

1. Introduction

Giardiasis is the intestinal infection caused by *Giardia lamblia* (also known as *Giardia intestinalis* or *Giardia duodenalis*). *G. lamblia* is a unicellular eukaryotic protozoan that was first described by Antonie van Leeuwenhoek in 1681—in his own stool sample [1]. For decades, it was considered of uncertain pathogenicity but now is recognized as common causes of diarrheal disease worldwide. Its clinical significance was broadly accepted after many symptomatic cases of giardiasis were diagnosed and reported among visitors to the Soviet Union in the early 1970s. Since then, giardiasis has been reported as responsible for many outbreaks throughout the world.

The epidemiology of giardiasis still is a matter of great discussion. From the original debates around its pathogenicity to the later ones about its speciation and biology, *G. lamblia* has proven to be an enigmatic and interesting organism [2]. Although giardiasis is currently recognized as one of the main causes of diarrheal disease and a leading cause of death and illness among children under 5 years old in developing countries [3], the long-term impact of pediatric giardiasis remains unclear. Recent cohort studies have confirmed a high prevalence of persistent, subclinical giardiasis and its association with growth shortfalls [4], but such evidence has not been consistently reported in the literature.

Commonly, giardiasis prevalence among poor populations is reported as very high, and when the infection became chronic, it has been associated also with malnutrition and cognitive deficits [5]. In developed countries, giardiasis represents the leading cause of traveler's diarrhea and is frequently reported among citizens that traveled to developing countries and expose themselves to untreated water from lakes, streams, and swimming pools [6–8]. These and other epidemiologic characteristics of giardiasis will be discussed in detail in this chapter based on the classical and latest literature.

2. Etiologic agent

G. lamblia is a parasitic protozoan of the order *Retortomonadida* that alternates between trophozoites and cysts forms within its life cycle, stages responsible for the clinical illness, and the transmission of the disease, respectively. Under the light microscope, trophozoites appear actively swimming and with its characteristically teardrop (viewed dorsoventrally) or spoon (viewed from the side) shaped, measuring 10–20 μm by 5–15 μm by 2–4 μm, containing four pairs of flagella, two identical nuclei, with a convex dorsum and a ventral disc that acts as a suction cup to facilitate attachment of the organism to the small bowel villi (**Figure 1A**). On high-quality slides, the parasite movement shows "falling leave mobility" and resembles a human face because of the positions of the median bodies, nuclei, and axonemes. Uncharacteristically *Giardia* trophozoites lack definable Golgi, peroxisomes, and true mitochondria, but have a menant mitosome. Trophozoites divide by binary fission, and cyst develops as feces dehydrated in transiting to the large bowel.

Microscopically, *Giardia* cysts look oval shaped, measures about 11–14 by 7–10 μm, contains four nuclei (mature cyst)—usually situated at one end—and curved median bodies and linear axonemes (**Figure 1B** and **C**). During the process of encystment, which can be observed under the microscope, trophozoites initially become inactive, rounded, and increasingly refractile as encystment begins. Then, nuclear division (but not cytoplasmic) occurs to produce the quadrinucleate infectious cyst. *Giardia* cysts have a thick hyaline wall that protects them from environmental stressors such as the alkaline environment that characterize the small intestinal, water chlorination, high-altitude, or extreme temperatures such as in boiling water. Also, such strong protection allows cysts to survive in water up to 3 months [9]. Upon excystation in the small bowel, each cyst releases two trophozoites, which continue the life cycle.

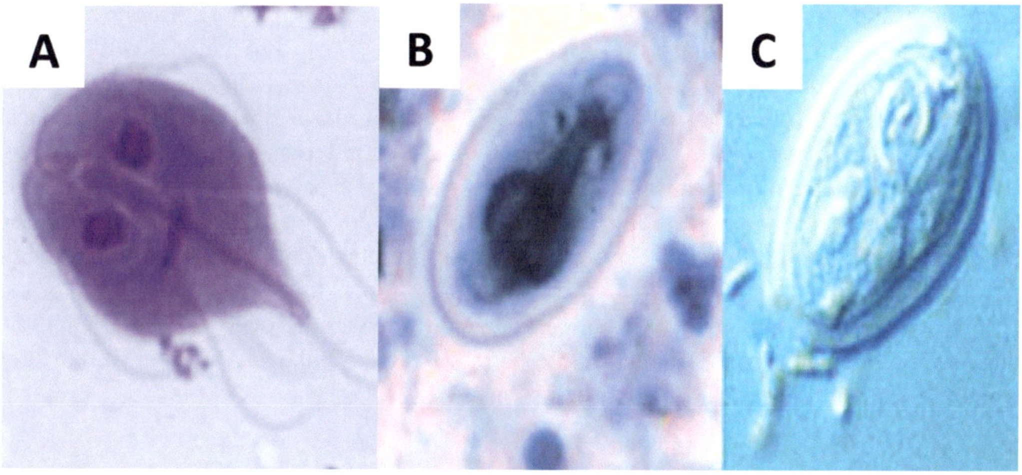

Figure 1. *Giardia lamblia*. Stained trophozoite (A) with its characteristic teardrop shape, binucleate structure, and four pairs of flagella clearly visible. Stained (B) and unstained (C) cysts with its characteristic median (parabasal) bodies and four nuclei. Images are some of the best public-domain light micrographs of *Giardia*, published by the National Institute of Infectious Diseases of Tokyo, Japan. Images were originally published at http://www.nih.go.jp/niid/ja/kansennohanashi/410-giardia.html.

Giardia species are currently classified in six species, which are distinguished based on its morphology and hosts: *Gracilinanus agilis* (amphibians), *G. lamblia* (mammals), *Giardia muris* (rodents), *Giardia psittaci*, and *Giardia ardeae* (both mainly in birds) (**Table 1**) [2]. Previously, many more species of *Giardia* were listed based only on microscopic and epidemiological criteria as well, but using molecular tests such as polymerase chain reaction (PCR), the list was shortened. Later on, genotyping studies confirmed that the species of *Giardia* could be classified in eight genetic groups (A–H): Groups A and B, which are found in humans and

Species	Hosts	Morphology
G. agilis	Amphibians	Longer and slender than *G. lamblia*, with a teardrop-shaped median body
G. ardeae	Herons and other birds	Similar to *G. lamblia*
G. lamblia	Mammals including humans, dogs, and some wild species	Teardrop shaped with claw-shaped median bodies
G. microti	Rodents, voles, and muskrats	Similar to *G. lamblia*
G. muris	Rodents	Shorter and rounder than *G. lamblia*, with small rounded median body
G. psittaci	Psittacine birds	Similar to *G. lamblia*

Adapted from Adam [2] and Caccio and Ryan [14].

Table 1. *Giardia* species.

many domestic animals and wildlife [10], and the host-specific groups C–H. Among the latest ones, groups C and D infect dogs, cats, coyotes, and wolves [11]; group E infects cattle, sheep, goats, pigs, water buffaloes, and mouflons [12]; group F infects cats [12]; group G infects rats [12]; and group H infects marine animals [13]. This classification could be of great clinical value given that in addition to many genetic differences found, these genotypes exhibit several relevant biologic differences also. In example, genotype B seems to be more pathogenic than genotype A in humans, although they appear to grow slower [14]. Contradictory, the genetics of parasites of the genus *Giardia* is still poorly understood. Furthermore, recent evidence has cast doubt the classical view of an asexually replicating organism in favor of the occurrence of meiosis and genetic exchange. Such game breaker discovery demanded that the whole population genetics of *Giardia* should be reevaluated to take into account the effect of recombination on *G. lamblia* species [14].

3. Life cycle

Life cycle begins with the infection by the ingestion of the cyst. Then the excystation continues, which starts at the stomach triggered by the exposure of the cyst to the gastric acid, the presence of bile and trypsin in the duodenum and/or the alkaline, protease-rich milieu, duodenum [2]. Excystation ends at the proximal small intestine where the emerging parasites (excyzoites) quickly transform into trophozoites that attach to the intestinal epithelial cells using the adhesive disc. The adhesive disc is essential for attachment and appears to play a major role in the virulence of *Giardia* [15]. Several disc-associated proteins have been identified using proteomics [16], and it is clear that the disc is an advanced cytoskeletal structure [17]. At the jejunum, the trophozoites start to encyst forming the wall that enables the parasite to survive outside the host for several weeks in cold water. This process is triggered by a particular composition of biliary secretions, possibly by a deprivation of cholesterol [18]. Regulatory factors are encystation-specific transcription factors, chromatin remodeling enzymes, and posttranslational modifications, which vary their expression in correlation with the variation of antigens on the parasite surface [19]. Finally, trophozoites and cysts are released with the stool, with cysts continuing the transmission of the disease when ingested by another host.

Reservoir hosts include humans, as well as a variety of animals, including cats, dogs, dairy cattle, beavers, and other farm, wild, and domesticated animals such as horses, pigs, cows, chinchillas, alpacas, lemurs, sheep, guinea pigs, monkeys, goats, and rats [20]. However, among all these animal hosts, only beavers, dogs, and humans have been implicated as a source of infection in different waterborne epidemics and outbreaks of giardiasis in humans. Additionally, it is important to highlight the key role of "reverse zoonotic transmission" (zooanthroponotic) in the epidemiology of *Giardia* infections, which means that humans have been identified as the source of infection for beavers, muskrats, and coyotes in the Unites States and Canada [21–23], muskoxen in the Canadian arctic [24], nonhuman primates (gorillas) and painted dogs in Africa [25], marsupials in Australia, house mice in remote islands [26], and marine mammals (seals) in various parts of the world [27].

Even in developed countries such as the United States, it is common to isolate *Giardia* cysts in the water reservoirs and unfiltered water supplies of major cities, the water supply that is not filtrated [28].

4. Incidence and burden of disease

G. lamblia has been consistently reported as one of the most common pathogens worldwide [29]. Due to high endemicity among humans, and domestic and wildlife animals, it is considered of public health and veterinary health importance [12]. Symptomatic infections have been reported by millions in Asia, Africa, and Latin America by the World Health Organization, which have estimated that it causes 183 million (confidence interval of 95%, 130–262 million) cases of giardiasis [30].

Worldwide, the incidence of Giardiasis has been estimated in 2.8×10^8 cases per year [31]. However, several epidemiological studies have reported that such rates could be significantly underestimated, with giardiasis prevalence rates ranging from 10 to 20% of the general population [32], from 10 to 50% in developing countries [33, 34], and from 2 to 5% in developed countries [35, 36]. This could be explained by the large fraction of asymptomatic carriers, which regardless of the absence of symptoms also contribute to the transmission of the diseases.

Giardiasis is a ubiquitous disease so it occurred across broad epidemiological contexts and with a broad range of distributions. On one side, in most developed countries such as the United Kingdom [37] and Germany [8], *Giardia* is mostly reported as a rare disease affecting travelers. Furthermore, in the countries such as the Unites States, where *Giardia* is continually under surveillance, *Giardia* has higher incidences (incidence rate ratios, 1.2–1.5) in counties with higher private well reliance compared to counties with lower well reliance [38]. On the other side, in most developing countries, *Giardia* has been associated with poor health hygiene, poor toilet training, overcrowding, and low socioeconomic status [39]. Furthermore, due to the high prevalence of *Giardia* among children, and its higher exposure to dogs in poor setting, it is believed that *Giardia* has developed zoonotic transmission. This possibility has been reported concordantly by genotyping and molecular studies from Mexico [40], Jamaica [41], and Cambodia [42].

The high prevalence of *Giardia* among children raised a major concern about their long-term impacts, which currently have been well documented and reported as more worrisome due to the association between persistent *Giardia* and children's growth [43]. *Giardia* infections can be detected repetitively in over 40% of children suggesting that persistent infections are common and associated with a damage of the intestinal permeability, which—independently of diarrhea—can lead to stunted growth. In fact, according to the results from the MAL-ED birth cohort study, the persistence of *Giardia* before 6 months of age was associated with a −0.29 (95% CI, −0.53 to −0.05) deficit in weight-for-age z score and −0.29 (95% CI, −0.64 to 0.07) deficit in length-for-age *z* score at 2 years [44].

5. Giardiasis epidemiology

The *Giardia* cysts are overall highly infectious, and as few as 10 cysts can cause an infection in an individual. Giardiasis prevalence rates have been reported consistently as high among young children from developing countries, with high rates of repeated infection even within the first year of life. However, many developed countries have many regions with endemic giardiasis or regular outbreaks. At these countries giardiasis outbreaks are particularly common during the summer months (likely due to recreational swimming exposure) or throughout the year around day-cares and nurseries, infecting children under 5 years old—and their caregivers—the most [45]. In fact, an investigation of 242 outbreaks, affecting 41,000 persons, reported that most outbreaks resulted from waterborne (74.8%), foodborne (15.7%), person-to-person (2.5%), and animal contact (1.2%) transmission, with waterborne outbreaks been that largest ones in terms of number of cases per outbreak [46].

Surveillance data cases have shown that giardiasis infects populations with a bimodal age distribution, peaking at ages 0–9 years and 45–49 years, without gender preferences [35], and within areas that are endemic, giardiasis commonly shows a seasonal pattern, with most cases occurring in the summer months due to a recent history of drinking untreated surface water and a history of swimming in a lake or pond or swimming in any natural body of fresh water [47]. Other risk factors that have been reported as associated to giardiasis in endemic areas include living in areas that use at-risk tap water (i.e., filtered or unfiltered surface water [48, 49] or unfiltered shallow well water [48]) or in rural areas [49].

One of the most common mechanisms of transmission of *Giardia* infections is a waterborne transmission but also can be transmitted by fecal-oral transmission with contaminated food or direct fecal-oral contact among family members, person-to-person contact, and sexual transmission (oral-anal contact). Although it is unclear which ones are clinically the most important, there is a common understanding about the populations at high risk of giardiasis, which include:

- diaper-age children who attend day-care centers [50, 51];
- adults that work in child-care organizations or day-care centers [52];
- institutionalized individuals [53];
- men who have sex with men [54];
- immunocompromised individuals (chronic variable immunodeficiency, hypogammaglobulinemia, HIV, immunosuppressed individuals, cystic fibrosis, and others) [55, 56]; and
- international travelers or any subject (hikers, campers, sportsman's adventures, and others) exposed to drinking untreated water from lakes, streams, and swimming pools [57].

Waterborne transmission is recognized as the most common transmission, with numerously documented outbreaks throughout the world [46, 58]. This includes the consumption of contaminated water from pools, rivers, or lakes, as well as from contaminated drinking water, either unpurified or inadequately purified. There have been multiple documented cases of cysts in the municipal water supply here in the United States, although such scenarios do not account for the vast majority of infections [35].

Foodborne transmission of *G. lamblia* is much less common than waterborne transmission, but there are many ways food can be fecally contaminated. For example, street food and any food prepared with the unclean hands of an infected subject could easily transmit giardiasis given a few cysts necessary to transmit the disease. Ingestion of 100 or more cysts is required to ensure infection in humans, but as few as 10 cysts have proven to be enough to infect a volunteer [59].

Fecal-oral transmission is also a significant mechanism of transmission and is the one responsible for the outbreaks in day-cares and nurseries. These outbreaks reflect the close contact between young children, who are significantly more likely to pass the parasite fecal-orally at day-cares than at home. For example, in the Netherlands, where around half of preschool children are cared for in day-care centers, a mean of 2.5 days a week, children at day-care centers are twice as likely to test positive to *G. lamblia* as their home-care counterparts [45], infecting around 4.2% of them [60].

Sexual transmission of *Giardia* is now a very well described form of oral-anal transmission and fecal-oral transmission among men who have sex with men. Currently, there exist a large body of publications that have led to improving our understanding of giardiasis as a sexually transmitted infection. According to these studies, prevalence rates of giardiasis among men who have sex with men range from 2 to 30% [61]. Although giardiasis is not a major cause of AIDS-associated diarrhea, the prevalence of giardiasis, as well as the chronicity of symptoms, is greater in patients with AIDS, especially in developing countries [62]. Overall, every immunocompromised group, like AIDS patients, is recognized as more susceptible to the development of chronic giardiasis [63].

To sum up, it is really important that healthcare providers consider *Giardia* as a differential diagnosis among high-risk populations that match giardiasis epidemiology, and if patients tested positive, it is really important that they provide patients with appropriate therapy and follow-up, as well as proper counseling to increase treatment compliance rate. And in the case of men who have sex with men, also encourage partner notification, and teach them strategies for preventing the transmission of this disease, including the discussion of the risk of enteric infections after oral-anal sexual contact.

Author details

Antonio Marty Quispe Gutiérrez[1,2]

Address all correspondence to: drantonioquispe@gmail.com

1 Johns Hopkins Bloomberg School of Public Health, International Health Department, Baltimore, Maryland, USA

2 Instituto de Evaluación de Tecnologías en Salud e Investigación (IETSI), EsSalud, Lima, Peru

References

[1] Ford BJ. The discovery of giardia. Microscope. 2005;**53**:147-153

[2] Adam RD. Biology of *Giardia lamblia*. Clinical Microbiology Review. 2001;**14**:447-475

[3] Kotloff KL, Nataro JP, Blackwelder WC, Nasrin D, Farag TH, Panchalingam S, Wu Y, Sow SO, Sur D, Breiman RF, Faruque AS, Zaidi AK, Saha D, Alonso PL, Tamboura B, Sanogo D, Onwuchekwa U, Manna B, Ramamurthy T, Kanungo S, Ochieng JB, Omore R, Oundo JO, Hossain A, Das SK, Ahmed S, Qureshi S, Quadri F, Adegbola RA, Antonio M, Hossain MJ, Akinsola A, Mandomando I, Nhampossa T, Acacio S, Biswas K, O'Reilly CE, Mintz ED, Berkeley LY, Muhsen K, Sommerfelt H, Robins-Browne RM, Levine MM. Burden and aetiology of diarrhoeal disease in infants and young children in developing countries (the Global Enteric Multicenter Study, GEMS): A prospective, case-control study. Lancet. 2013;**382**:209-222

[4] Bartelt LA, Platts-Mills JA. Giardia: A pathogen or commensal for children in high-prevalence settings? Current Opinion in Infectious Disease. 2016;**29**:502-507

[5] Fraser D, Bilenko N, Deckelbaum RJ, Dagan R, El-On J, Naggan L. *Giardia lamblia* carriage in Israeli Bedouin infants: Risk factors and consequences. Clinical Infectious Disease. 2000;**30**:419-424

[6] Brodsky RE, Spencer HC Jr., Schultz MG. Giardiasis in American travelers to the Soviet Union. Journal of Infectious Disease. 1974;**130**:319-323

[7] Lopez CE, Juranek DD, Sinclair SP, Schultz MG. Giardiasis in American travelers to Madeira Island, Portugal. American Journal of Tropical Medicine and Hygiene. 1978;**27**:1128-1132

[8] Jelinek T, Loscher T. Epidemiology of giardiasis in German travelers. Journal of Travel Medicine. 2000;**7**:70-73

[9] Wolfe MS. Giardiasis. Clinical Microbiology Review. 1992;**5**:93-100

[10] Monis PT, Caccio SM, Thompson RC. Variation in giardia: Towards a taxonomic revision of the genus. Trends in Parasitology. 2009;**25**:93-100

[11] Caccio SM, Thompson RC, McLauchlin J, Smith HV. Unravelling *Cryptosporidium* and giardia epidemiology. Trends in Parasitology. 2005;**21**:430-437

[12] Feng Y, Xiao L. Zoonotic potential and molecular epidemiology of *Giardia* species and giardiasis. Clinical Microbiology Review. 2011;**24**:110-140

[13] Lasek-Nesselquist E, Welch DM, Sogin ML. The identification of a new *Giardia duodenalis* assemblage in marine vertebrates and a preliminary analysis of *G. duodenalis* population biology in marine systems. Int Journal of Parasitology. 2010;**40**:1063-1074

[14] Caccio SM, Ryan U. Molecular epidemiology of giardiasis. Molecular and Biochemical Parasitology. 2008;**160**:75-80

[15] Dawson SC. An insider's guide to the microtubule cytoskeleton of giardia. Cellular Microbiology. 2010;**12**:588-598

[16] Hagen KD, Hirakawa MP, House SA, Schwartz CL, Pham JK, Cipriano MJ, De La Torre MJ, Sek AC, Du G, Forsythe BM, Dawson SC. Novel structural components of the ventral disc and lateral crest in *Giardia intestinalis*. PLoS Neglected Tropical Disease. 2011;**5**:e1442

[17] Brown JR, Schwartz CL, Heumann JM, Dawson SC, Hoenger A. A detailed look at the cytoskeletal architecture of the *Giardia lamblia* ventral disc. Journal of Structural Biology. 2016;**194**:38-48

[18] Lujan HD, Mowatt MR, Byrd LG, Nash TE. Cholesterol starvation induces differentiation of the intestinal parasite *Giardia lamblia*. Proceedings of National Academy Science United States of America. 1996;**93**:7628-7633

[19] Einarsson E, Troell K, Hoeppner MP, Grabherr M, Ribacke U, Svard SG. Coordinated changes in gene expression throughout encystation of *Giardia intestinalis*. PLoS Neglected Tropical Disease. 2016;**10**:e0004571

[20] Gilman RH, Brown KH, Visvesvara GS, Mondal G, Greenberg B, Sack RB, Brandt F, Khan MU. Epidemiology and serology of *Giardia lamblia* in a developing country: Bangladesh. Transactions of the Royal Society of Tropical Medicine and Hygiene. 1985;**79**:469-473

[21] Trout JM, Santin M, Fayer R. Giardia and Cryptosporidium species and genotypes in coyotes (*Canis latrans*). Journal of Zoo and Wildlife Medicine. 2006;**37**:141-144

[22] Thompson RC, Colwell DD, Shury T, Appelbee AJ, Read C, Njiru Z, Olson ME. The molecular epidemiology of Cryptosporidium and Giardia infections in coyotes from Alberta, Canada, and observations on some cohabiting parasites. Veterinary Parasitology. 2009;**159**:167-170

[23] Fayer R, Santin M, Trout JM, DeStefano S, Koenen K, Kaur T. Prevalence of Microsporidia, Cryptosporidium spp., and Giardia spp. in beavers (*Castor canadensis*) in Massachusetts. Journal of Zoo and Wildlife Medicine. 2006;**37**:492-497

[24] Kutz SJ, Thompson RA, Polley L, Kandola K, Nagy J, Wielinga CM, Elkin BT. Giardia assemblage A: Human genotype in muskoxen in the Canadian Arctic. Parasit Vectors. 2008;**1**:32

[25] Graczyk TK, Bosco-Nizeyi J, Ssebide B, Thompson RC, Read C, Cranfield MR. Anthropozoonotic *Giardia duodenalis* genotype (assemblage) a infections in habitats of free-ranging human-habituated gorillas, Uganda. Journal of Parasitology. 2002;**88**:905-909

[26] Moro D, Lawson MA, Hobbs RP, Thompson RC. Pathogens of house mice on arid Boullanger Island and subantarctic Macquarie Island, Australia. Journal of Wildlife Disease. 2003;**39**:762-771

[27] Appelbee AJ, Thompson RC, Olson ME. Giardia and Cryptosporidium in mammalian wildlife—current status and future needs. Trends in Parasitology. 2005;**21**:370-376

[28] Beer KD, Gargano JW, Roberts VA, Hill VR, Garrison LE, Kutty PK, Hilborn ED, Wade TJ, Fullerton KE, Yoder JS. Surveillance for waterborne disease outbreaks associated with drinking water—United States, 2011-2012. MMWR Morbidity and Mortality Weekly Report. 2015;**64**:842-848

[29] Pires SM, Fischer-Walker CL, Lanata CF, Devleesschauwer B, Hall AJ, Kirk MD, Duarte AS, Black RE, Angulo FJ. Aetiology-specific estimates of the global and regional incidence and mortality of diarrhoeal diseases commonly transmitted through food. PLoS One. 2015;**10**:e0142927

[30] Torgerson PR, Devleesschauwer B, Praet N, Speybroeck N, Willingham AL, Kasuga F, Rokni MB, Zhou XN, Fevre EM, Sripa B, Gargouri N, Furst T, Budke CM, Carabin H, Kirk MD, Angulo FJ, Havelaar A, de Silva N. World Health Organization estimates of the global and regional disease burden of 11 foodborne parasitic diseases, 2010: A data synthesis. PLoS Medicine. 2015;**12**:e1001920

[31] Lane S, Lloyd D. Current trends in research into the waterborne parasite Giardia. Critical Reviews in Microbiology. 2002;**28**:123-147

[32] Gbakima AA. Intestinal parasitic infections and swamp development in Sierra Leone. African Journal of Health Sciences. 1994;**1**:175-178

[33] Savioli L, Smith H, Thompson A. Giardia and Cryptosporidium join the 'neglected diseases initiative'. Trends in Parasitology. 2006;**22**:203-208

[34] Daly ER, Roy SJ, Blaney DD, Manning JS, Hill VR, Xiao L, Stull JW. Outbreak of giardiasis associated with a community drinking-water source. Epidemiology and Infection. 2010;**138**:491-500

[35] Painter JE, Gargano JW, Collier SA, Yoder JS. Centers for Disease C, Prevention. Giardiasis surveillance—United States, 2011-2012. MMWR. 2015;64(3):15-25

[36] Yoder JS, Gargano JW, Wallace RM, Beach MJ, Centers for Disease C, Prevention. Giardiasis surveillance--United States, 2009-2010. MMWR Surveillance Summary. 2012; **61**:13-23

[37] Takaoka K, Gourtsoyannis Y, Hart JD, Armstrong M, Daniel A, Mewse E, Phillips D, Bailey RL. Incidence rate and risk factors for giardiasis and strongyloidiasis in returning UK travellers. Journal of Travel Medicine. 2016;23(5):1-6

[38] Schnell K, Collier S, Derado G, Yoder J, Gargano JW. Giardiasis in the United States—an epidemiologic and geospatial analysis of county-level drinking water and sanitation data, 1993-2010. Journal of Water and Health. 2016;**14**:267-279

[39] Rodriguez-Morales AJ, Granados-Alvarez S, Escudero-Quintero H, Vera-Polania F, Mondragon-Cardona A, Diaz-Quijano FA, Sosa-Valencia L, Lozada-Riascos CO, Escobedo AA, Liseth O, Haque U. Estimating and mapping the incidence of giardiasis in Colombia, 2009-2013. International Journal of Infectious Disease. 2016;**49**:204-209

[40] Garcia-Cervantes PC, Baez-Flores ME, Delgado-Vargas F, Ponce-Macotela M, Nawa Y, De-la-Cruz-Otero MD, Martinez-Gordillo MN, Diaz-Camacho SP. *Giardia duodenalis* genotypes among schoolchildren and their families and pets in urban and rural areas of Sinaloa, Mexico. Journal of Infection in Developing Countries. 2017;**11**:180-187

[41] Lee MF, Cadogan P, Eytle S, Copeland S, Walochnik J, Lindo JF. Molecular epidemiology and multilocus sequence analysis of potentially zoonotic Giardia spp. from humans and dogs in Jamaica. Parasitology Research. 2017;**116**:409-414

[42] Moore CE, Elwin K, Phot N, Seng C, Mao S, Suy K, Kumar V, Nader J, Bousfield R, Perera S, Bailey JW, Beeching NJ, Day NP, Parry CM, Chalmers RM. Molecular characterization of Cryptosporidium Species and *Giardia duodenalis* from symptomatic Cambodian children. PLoS Neglected Tropical Diseases. 2016;**10**:e0004822

[43] Kosek MN, Investigators M-EN. Causal pathways from enteropathogens to environmental enteropathy: Findings from the MAL-ED birth cohort study. EBioMedicine. 2017;**18**:109-117

[44] Rogawski ET, Bartelt LA, Platts-Mills JA, Seidman JC, Samie A, Havt A, Babji S, Trigoso DR, Qureshi S, Shakoor S, Haque R, Mduma E, Bajracharya S, Gaffar SMA, Lima AAM, Kang G, Kosek MN, Ahmed T, Svensen E, Mason C, Bhutta ZA, Lang DR, Gottlieb M, Guerrant RL, Houpt ER, Bessong PO. Determinants and impact of Giardia infection in the first 2 years of life in the MAL-ED birth cohort. Journal of the Pediatric Infectious Diseases Society. 2017;**6**:153-160

[45] Pijnacker R, Mughini-Gras L, Heusinkveld M, Roelfsema J, van Pelt W, Kortbeek T. Different risk factors for infection with *Giardia lamblia* assemblages A and B in children attending day-care centres. European Journal of Clinical Microbiology and Infectious Disease. 2016;**35**:2005-2013

[46] Adam EA, Yoder JS, Gould LH, Hlavsa MC, Gargano JW. Giardiasis outbreaks in the United States, 1971-2011. Epidemiology and Infection. 2016;**144**:2790-2801

[47] Dennis DT, Smith RP, Welch JJ, Chute CG, Anderson B, Herndon JL, von Reyn CF. Endemic giardiasis in New Hampshire: A case-control study of environmental risks. Journal of Infectious Disease. 1993;**167**:1391-1395

[48] Gagnon F, Duchesne JF, Levesque B, Gingras S, Chartrand J. Risk of giardiasis associated with water supply in an endemic context. International Journal of Environmental Health Research. 2006;**16**:349-359

[49] Odoi A, Martin SW, Michel P, Holt J, Middleton D, Wilson J. Determinants of the geographical distribution of endemic giardiasis in Ontario, Canada: A spatial modelling approach. Epidemiology and Infection. 2004;**132**:967-976

[50] Duffy TL, Montenegro-Bethancourt G, Solomons NW, Belosevic M, Clandinin MT. Prevalence of giardiasis in children attending semi-urban daycare centres in Guatemala and comparison of 3 giardia detection tests. Journal of Health, Population and Nutrition. 2013;**31**:290-293

[51] Nunez FA, Hernandez M, Finlay CM. Longitudinal study of giardiasis in three day care centres of Havana City. Acta Tropica. 1999;**73**:237-242

[52] Boreham PF, Shepherd RW. Giardiasis in child-care centres. Medical Journal of Australia. 1984;**141**:263

[53] Mascarini LM, Donalisio MR. Giardiasis and cryptosporidiosis in children institutionalized at daycare centers in the state of Sao Paulo. Revista da Sociedade Brasileira de Medicina Tropical. 2006;**39**:577-579

[54] Beltrami JF, Shouse RL, Blake PA. Trends in infectious diseases and the male to female ratio: Possible clues to changes in behavior among men who have sex with men. AIDS Education and Prevention. 2005;**17**:49-59

[55] Abaza SM, Makhlouf LM, el-Shewy KA, el-Moamly AA. Intestinal opportunistic parasites among different groups of immunocompromised hosts. Journal of the Egyptian Society of Parasitology. 1995;**25**:713-727

[56] Cruz I, Ricardo JL, Nunes JF, Serras AC, Porto MT, Lopes JM, Veloso FT, Freitas J. Giardia and immune deficiency. American Journal of Gastroenterology. 1991;**86**:1554-1555

[57] Holtan NR. Giardiasis. A crimp in the life-style of campers, travelers, and others. Postgraduate Medicine Journal. 1988;**83**:54-6, 59-61

[58] Guzman-Herrador B, Carlander A, Ethelberg S, Freiesleben de Blasio B, Kuusi M, Lund V, Lofdahl M, MacDonald E, Nichols G, Schonning C, Sudre B, Tronnberg L, Vold L, Semenza JC, Nygard K. Waterborne outbreaks in the Nordic countries, 1998 to 2012. EuroSurveillance. 2015;**20**

[59] Rendtorff RC, Holt CJ. The experimental transmission of human intestinal protozoan parasites. IV. Attempts to transmit Entamoeba coli and *Giardia lamblia* cysts by water. American Journal of Hygiene. 1954;60(3):327-338

[60] Enserink R, Scholts R, Bruijning-Verhagen P, Duizer E, Vennema H, de Boer R, Kortbeek T, Roelfsema J, Smit H, Kooistra-Smid M, van Pelt W. High detection rates of enteropathogens in asymptomatic children attending day care. PLoS One. 2014;**9**:e89496

[61] Escobedo AA, Almirall P, Alfonso M, Cimerman S, Chacin-Bonilla L. Sexual transmission of giardiasis: A neglected route of spread? Acta Tropica. 2014;**132**:106-111

[62] Manatsathit S, Tansupasawasdikul S, Wanachiwanawin D, Setawarin S, Suwanagool P, Prakasvejakit S, Leelakusolwong S, Eampokalap B, Kachintorn U. Causes of chronic diarrhea in patients with AIDS in Thailand: A prospective clinical and microbiological study. Journal of Gastroenterology. 1996;**31**:533-537

[63] Espelage W, an der Heiden M, Stark K, Alpers K. Characteristics and risk factors for symptomatic *Giardia lamblia* infections in Germany. BMC Public Health. 2010;**10**:41

Chapter 3

Malabsorption in Giardiasis

Amornnivit Kanokwanvimol

Additional information is available at the end of the chapter

http://dx.doi.org/10.5772/intechopen.70806

Abstract

Giardia intestinalis is a flagellated parasite and is regarded as the most common cause of protozoan-associated diarrhoea worldwide. The organisms can be found in 80% of raw water supplies from lakes, streams and ponds and as many as 15% filtered water samples. *Giardia* intestinalis can be found worldwide including both temperate and tropical regions and can cause asymptomatic colonisation or acute or chronic diarrhoea illness. The symptoms vary from vague abdominal discomfort or severe abdominal pain, diarrhoea and weight loss. It is believed that these symptoms are a result of giardiasis-associated malabsorption syndrome, although the pathophysiology underlying intestinal disturbances remains incompletely understood. Interestingly, intestinal malabsorption is a result of epithelial dysfunction that shares similarities with those observed in other enteric disorders such as bacteria enteritis, Crohn's disease and celiac disease. Numerous other mechanisms of intestinal malabsorption have been postulated such as immunologic reactions, altered gut motility and fluid hypersecretion via adenylate cyclase activity. In this chapter, we will go through each mechanism of malabsorption associated with giardiasis and the consequences of this to the patients.

Keywords: intestinal malabsorption, giardiasis, epithelia, injury, growth retardation, chronic diarrhoea

1. Introduction

Giardia infection is a common intestinal infection worldwide [1, 2]. The worldwide incidence was estimated at 2.8×10^8 infection per year [3]. In the industrialised world, overall prevalence rates are 2–5%. In developing world, infection starts as early as in the infant year and is the major cause of childhood diarrhoea. Prevalence rates of 15–20% in children under 10 years are common [2, 4]. In Thailand, the prevalence of giardiasis ranges from 1.25 to 37.7% [5]. The incidence varies depending on age, living conditions, personal hygiene and environment sanitation. Despite the high prevalence of the infection, physicians often neglect to add giardiasis as one of the differential diagnosis in patients present with chronic diarrhoea. This is due to the lack of expertise in many of our public hospitals.

Patients who are infected with *Giardia* intestinalis have symptoms ranging from asymptomatic to severe chronic diarrhoea. The pathogenesis of malabsorption syndrome–related chronic diarrhoea is not fully understood; however, many theories such as epithelial dysfunction, immunologic reactions, altered gut motility and fluid hypersecretion have been postulated.

Giardiasis can lead to grown retardation in children and severe malnutrition in adult patients. Patients can also present with protein energy malnutrition, vitamin A deficiency and iron deficiency anaemia. A cross sectional study in Malaysia including 281 children aged 2–15 years showed that 56.5% of the infected children have significantly underweight, while 61.3% have growth retardations [6].

2. Pathophysiology of malabsorption

2.1. Electrolyte transport abnormality

Giardiasis causes malabsorption of glucose, sodium and water and reduces disaccharidase activity due to loss of absorptive surface area [6]. Recent report also suggests that this parasite alters chloride secretory response in human colonic cells in vitro, as well as in murine models [7]. Moreover, study by Troeger et al. proved that in addition to malabsorption, chronic giardiasis may cause chloride hypersecretion in human [8]. Therefore, combinations of malabsorption and electrolyte transport abnormality are responsible for fluid accumulation in the intestinal lumen. The reasons behind these abnormalities remain poorly understood; however, multiple studies and reports suggest that parasite products may break the epithelial barrier. This activated T lymphocyte causing brush border to retract, which in turn leads to the disaccharidase deficiencies and epithelial malabsorption responsible for watery diarrhoea (**Figure 1**) [9, 10]. In fact, epithelial cells dysfunctions and disaccharide deficiencies are medicated by CD8+ T cells, whereas CD4+ T cells contribute to parasite clearance [11, 12]. Moreover, findings that athymic mice infected with *Giardia* do not exhibit microvillus injury and dysfunction despite the presence of live parasites refute the hypothesis that intestinal malfunction solely results from trophozoite attachment or parasite virulence factors [8, 11, 12].

2.2. Role of parasite virulence factors

Stain-dependent activation of enterocyte apoptosis and epithelial dysfunction induced by *Giardia* may occur in the absence of any other cell types, and small intestinal permeability returns to baseline once *Giardia* is cleared [13]. Virulence factors in *Giardia* and its effect are currently under intensive research. Giardia is thought to express a certain surface glycoprotein able to induce fluid accumulation in the intestine. Moreover, this organism is known to produce variety of potentially toxic substances such as proteinase and lectins that maybe responsible for direct epithelia injury [14, 15]. Much genomic studies are still needed to identify *Giardia's* enterotoxin and ability of *Giardia*'s proteinase to activate host receptors; however, multiple studies have reported that proteinase along with *Giardia* enterotoxins are an important virulence

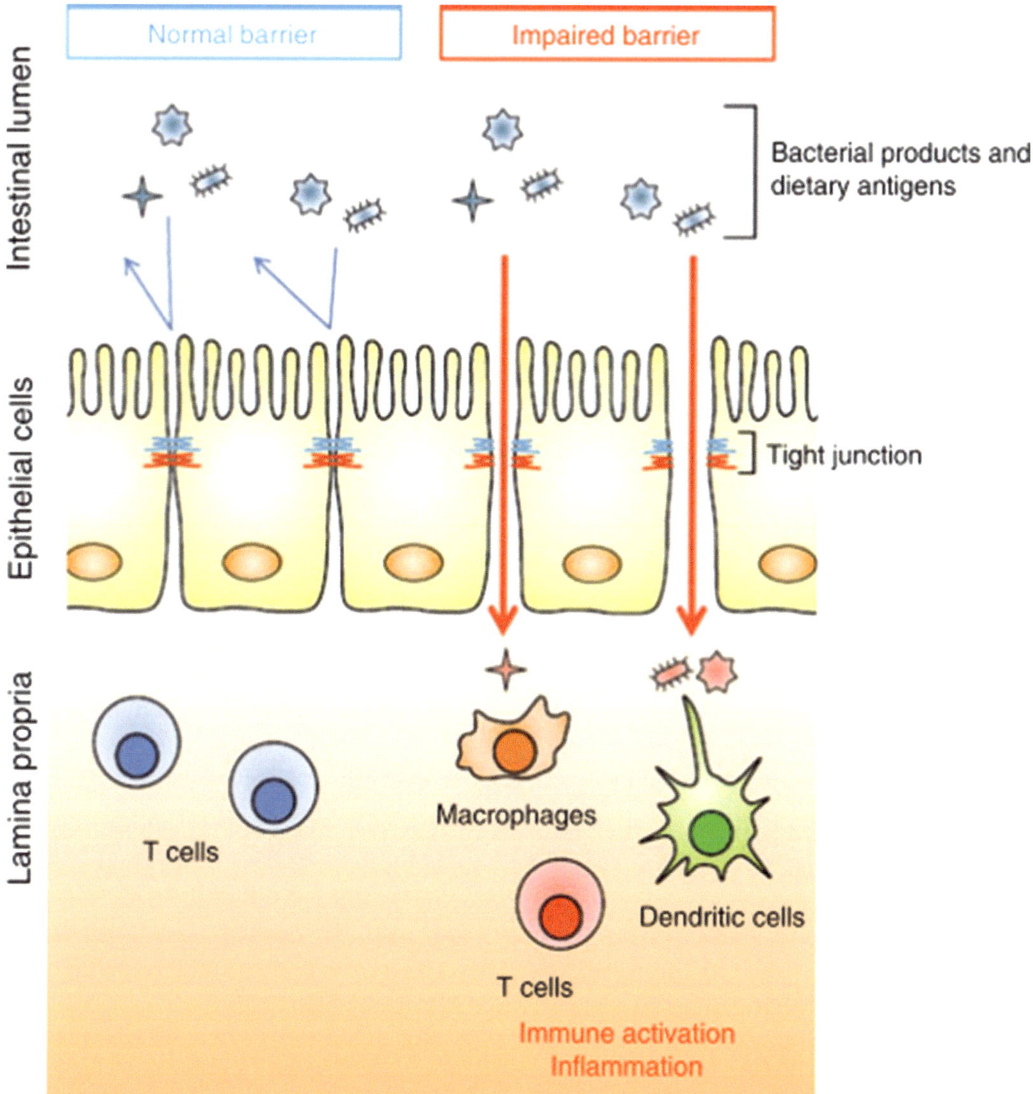

Figure 1. Impaired epithelial tight junctions as a result from attachment of *Giardia*'s trophozoite causing activations of immune response by influx of bacterial products leading to activation of T cells causing injury to brush boarder leading to malabsorption and diarrhoea.

factors in many organisms including *Giardia*. Proteinase-activated receptors are member of class G-protein coupled signalling receptors that can modulate enterocyte apoptosis and increase intestinal permeability [16]. **Table 1** shows example of *Giardia* major virulence factor [17].

2.3. Other possible pathophysiology of giardiasis

As in the case with other enteropathogens, induction of apoptosis in enterocytes by *Giardia* is the key components of the pathophysiology of giardiasis [18, 19]. Enterocytes apoptosis in giardiasis

Function	Virulence factor
Attachment	Colonisation and attachment to intestinal endothelium is by the ventral adhesive disc and surface lecithin
Circumvention of the natural factors of the intestinal lumen	Re-localization by flagellar motility allows further colonisation. Protective factors such as variant-specific surface protein (VSP) protect *Giardia* from luminal proteases
Antigenic variation	*Giardia* is cleared from the body by IgA directed clearance. This is protected by VSP
Alteration of host innate defences	Down regulate epithelial production of nitric oxide by releasing arginine deaminase
Anti-inflammatory modifications	Unknown trophozoite products have anti-inflammatory roles
Survival in stomach acid and the external environment	Differentiation into cysts

IgA, immunoglobulin A; VSP, variant-specific surface protein.

Table 1. The major virulence factors of *Giardia* spp. *Giardia* is a complex organism; they produce complex enterotoxin and proteinase causing epithelial cell damage.

is Caspase 3, Caspase 9 dependent [20]. The reasons behind the activations of these proteins, which play crucial roles in apoptosis, still have not been fully understood. However, it is believed that both host and parasite factors modulate the activation of these proteins, although the exact mechanism is still not known. Interestingly, Giardia's trophozoites may halt enterocytes cell-cycle progression by consumption of arginine and upregulation of cell-cycle inhibitory genes [21].

Other possible key pathophysiology of giardiasis is *Giardia*-induced epithelial bush boarder microvilli shortening. This leads to symptoms of maldigestion and malabsorption such as diarrhoea. The factor contribute to microvilli shortening is still not fully validated; however, it was postulated that parasite's toxins may play a key role in the development of this abnormality. This is very similar to "protease" which was released in patients with bacterial overgrowth causing villi shortening and malabsorption syndrome [22].

Giardia infections tend to be self-limiting in immune-competent patient. A recent study in Brazilian children suggests that symptoms are less severe during re-infection. This supports the previous hypothesis that, during the primary infection, the immunity develops leading to less severe symptoms [23]. Patients who are immunodeficiency or have common variable immune deficiency such as Bruton's X-linked agammaglobulinema are prone to chronic giardiasis. This finding confirms the importance of immune system in giardiasis [24].

3. Symptoms and sign of chronic infection with giardiasis

Chronic infection is particularly important in children as it may cause malabsorption leading to growth retardation. There are reports of small intestinal villous atrophy especially in children. It is important at this stage to exclude coeliac sprue on gastrointestinal immunodeficiency syndrome for the correct diagnosis to be made [25].

Other symptoms include:

3.1. Chronic diarrhoea

A small number of people develop acute explosive watery diarrhoea, foul flatus, abdominal cramps and vomiting. These symptoms usually last 3–4 days before subacute symptoms develop. Symptoms of chronic infection including chronic diarrhoea, anorexia and weight loss occur as much as 66% of the infected individuals [1]. Chronic sporadic diarrhoea may continue for months, and post-infected lactase deficiency also presented in 5–40% of cases [1].

Stools of the infected individuals become more mushy, malodourous and greasy. Watery diarrhoea may alternate with soft stools or even constipation. Steatorrhea is a common finding in patients who have malabsorption syndrome.

3.2. Function gastrointestinal disorder

FGID represents a group of disorders characterised by recurring gastrointestinal symptoms. IBS and functional dyspepsia are best describing FGID. There are multiple reports of post-infectious IBS following salmonella, campylobacter infections. These usually follow episodes of acute gastroenteritis. Interestingly, recent reports suggest that individuals who are infected with *Giardia duodenalis* develop post-infectious IBS symptoms without parasitic load [26]. Irritable bowel syndrome (IBS) characterised by abdominal discomfort associated with altered bowel habit with no abnormality in routine diagnostic test. One common theory that has been postulated is that these symptoms develop following episodes of acute gastroenteritis. This explains the persisting symptoms of chronic diarrhoea and abdominal pain despite parasite clearance [27]. The risk of developing IBS increases six-fold after gastrointestinal infection as shown from multiple recent meta-analyses. This is interesting because these risks could remain elevated for at least 2–3 years post-infection. Moreover, it is estimated that 7–31% of patients with gastroenteritis go on to develop post-infectious IBS [27, 28]. Risk factors of developing IBS in this situation include longer duration of symptoms, younger age and female gender. The exact mechanisms of post-infectious IBS is still not known; however, there are reports that suggest that it associates with increase intestinal permeability, increase gut motility and increase number of enterochromaffin cells leading to persistent intestinal inflammation, which is characterised by increase T lymphocytes, mask cells and inflammatory cytokines [29, 30].

3.3. Other gastrointestinal symptoms

Report suggests that symptoms of lactase intolerance such as excessive flatus, abdominal bloating and diarrhoea can occur as a consequence of giardiasis. These patients will not be able to take milk, cheese or any products that contain lactose. It may take up to 1 month following the clearance of the parasite until the body return to normal state.

4. Extraintestinal manifestation of giardiasis and long-term consequences

4.1. Nutritional consequences

In combination with diarrhoea, giardiasis leads to iron deficiency anaemia, micronutrient deficiencies, protein-energy malnutrition, growth and cognitive retardation and malabsorption [31]. Studies from Peru and Brazil found that diarrhoea disease occurring in the first 2 years of life negatively correlates with verbal fluency, cognitive function and may lead to long-term growth failure [32]. Growth failure is assessed by anthropometric indices such as height for weight, height for age and weight for age. Interestingly, the prevalence of giardiasis is higher among children between 6 months and 5 years in developing country as compare to industrialised country [33]. Therefore, it has long been linked optimum health of children, socio-economic status, socio-cultural and environmental factors (**Table 2**).

4.2. Failure to thrive

Failure to thrive (FTT) is the term used when a child present with a rate of weight gain that is significantly below the expected weight from children of the same age, sex and ethnicity [34]. Common causes of FTT are inadequate food intake, inadequate food absorption, or maldigestion of nutrients and excessive loss of nutrient [34]. There is a strong association between *Giardia* infection and malnutrition, wasting and stunting [31–33]. Malabsorption, maldigestion and malnutrition due to giardiasis have been shown to affect anthropomorphic factors as well as calories intake during childhood especially in the second year of life [31]. Researchers now

Post-infectious consequence	Speculated mechanism involved
Ocular pathologies	Speculated involvement of toxic metabolite produced by the parasite.
Arthritis	Increase intestinal permeability leads to increase bacteria in synovial fluid joint.
Allergy	Alteration of antigen uptake due to dysfunction of the intestinal barrier.
Hypokalemic myopathy	Loss of potassium related to diarrhoea, impaired nutrient and electrolyte absorption
Failure to thrive	Inadequate food intake, reduced nutrients absorption, excessive utilisation of energy, steatorrhea, maldigestion, malabsorption
Stunting	Nutritional status, sanitary, socio-economic conditions, loss of intestinal surface area, maldigestion, malabsorption
Impaired cognitive function	Chronic malnutrition and stunting following G. duodenalis
Post infectious irritable bowel syndrome	Microscopic duodenal inflammation. Interaction host-gastrointestinal microbiota. Increased T-cells and Mast-cells
Cancer	Still need further research

Table 2. Extraintestinal and long-term complication of giardiasis.

develop key predictors of FTT and growth disturbance such as severity of diarrhoea diseases and duration of infection episodes [35]. Of note, vitamin deficiencies such as vitamin A, B1, B3, B6 and B12 are common reasons behind grown stunt in children infected with giardiasis.

4.3. Cancer

Multiple reports have described pancreatic cancer with pancreatic giardiasis. However, the relationship of these remains unknown. The coexistence of these two diseases may prompt further research into mechanism of carcinogenesis in giardiasis [36]. Interestingly, *Giardia's* trophozoite is usually found in proximal small intestine, but they can be identified in stomach, distal small bowel, and caecum, and there are reports of pancreatic infection with giardiasis [37].

4.4. Impair cognitive function

Cognitive functions are important especially in the first 2 years of life, as there is rapid brain growth and maturation. Nutrition, infection and other environmental factors have been found to affect neuroplasticity and have long-lasting effect in developing children [38]. One of the most important causes of brain development abnormality is malnutrition. Micronutrients deficiencies (such as iodine) and iron deficiency have been found to cause impairment in cognitive function in children [38]. The complex interaction among malnutrition, diarrheal disease and environmental factors such as low socioeconomic status and education makes it extremely difficult to determine the exact reason for cognitive impairment [39, 40]. However, chronic malnutrition and stunting during infancy secondary to giardiasis have been associated with poor cognitive functions [39–41]. Furthermore, diarrheal disease during early childhood was found to impair visual-motor co-ordination, auditory, short-term memory and cortical cognitive functions [40].

There are studies that associate *Giardia* with poor language cognition and impair psychomotor development [31]. These studies also demonstrate a role for nutrient malabsorption and micronutrient deficiencies such as zinc, iron, or vitamin (A and B12) in human and in animals [40–42]. It was widely known that significantly lower serum ferritin and iron affect psychomotor development, and this has been detected in patients with giardiasis [38]. Similarly, diarrheal disease due to giardiasis was linked to poor cognitive function by causing zinc and iron micronutrient deficiency, as well as defects in anti-oxidant system which can affect neuroplasticity [38]. Zinc supplements were found to decrease the rate of diarrhoea caused by giardiasis [43]. This issue remains complicated, and further investigation is needed to the reversal of cognitive impairment following micronutrient supplement or *giardia* clearance.

4.5. Muscular complications

Hypokalaemia myopathy has long been associated with coeliac disease, radiation enteritis and infections. Several cases of myopathy following hypokalaemia induced by giardiasis have been reported with both immunocompromised and immunocompetent patients [44]. This suggests that *giardia* can trigger muscular manifestations independently to the immune status of the host. During infection, potassium loss is related to number of bout of diarrhoea per day [44]. Hypokalaemia following bouts of diarrhoea is the trigger of transient myopathy.

In fact, after the resolve of diarrhoea, myopathy also improves. Main symptoms of these patients are proximal myopathy which is transient, but patients may have other co-morbid symptoms associated with hypokalaemia.

5. Diagnosis

5.1. History

To diagnose giardiasis, an expert microbiologist is required to identify giardia trophozoite in stool samples. Initial steps to diagnose malabsorption require extensive history and physical examinations. Duration of diarrhoea, stool characteristic and presentation of other symptoms such as poor night vision (vitamin A deficiency), pin and needles in both arms and legs (vitamin B6, B12 deficiency), poor cognitive functions, muscle wasting and significant weight lost suggest present of malabsorption. However, extensive history is still needed to exclude other differential diagnosis of chronic diarrhoea [45] (**Table 3**). History of travel especially to the endemic area of *giardia* helps increase suspicion for this infection.

Effective ways in history taking is to know the differential diagnosis of diarrhoea.

Other information that should be obtained is

1. Onset: gradual, sudden, congenital. Diarrhoea caused from malabsorption usually progressive in term of frequency and consistency.
2. Pattern: continuous or intermittent.
3. Iatrogenic factors such as drugs, radiation, tube feeding.
4. Systematic diseases such as endocrine (hypothyroidism, hypothyroidism), immunological diseases, and neoplasm.
5. Other associated symptoms such as abdominal pain (location, precipitating, aggravating, relieving factors).

Type of diarrhoea	Causes	Example
Secretory	Exogenous secretagogues	Enterotoxins (e.g., cholera)
	Endogenous secretagogues	Neuroendocrine tumours (e.g, carcinoid syndrome)
	Absence of ion transporter	Congenital chloridorrhea
	Loss of intestinal surface area	Intestinal resection, diffuse intestinal mucosal disease
	Intestinal ischemia	Diffuse mesenteric atherosclerosis
	Rapid intestinal transit	Intestinal hurry following vagotomy
Osmotic	Ingestion of poorly absorbed agent	Magnesium ingestion
	Reduced nutrient transport	Lactase deficiency

Table 3. Differential diagnosis of chronic diarrhoea [45].

http://dx.doi.org/10.5772/intechopen.70806

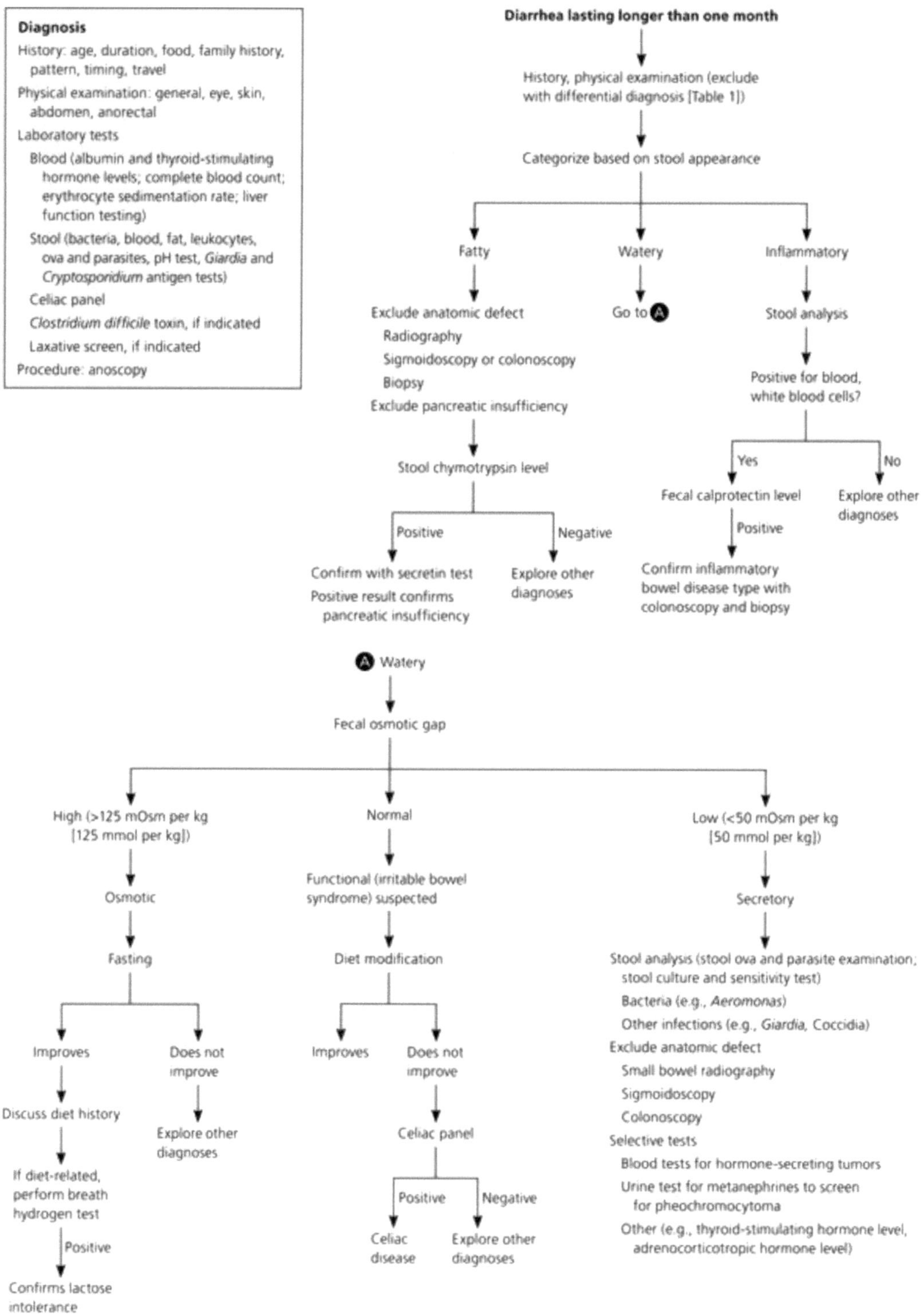

Figure 2. Diagnosis algorithm for chronic diarrhoea.

As **Table 3**, the initial step in the evaluation of chronic diarrhoea is to send stool off for assessment of stool osmotic gap. This allows the differentiation of chronic watery diarrhoea into secretory (faecal osmotic gap <50 mOsm per kg) and osmotic (faecal osmotic gap >125 mOsm per kg). Watery diarrhoea is likely osmotic because the symptoms caused by malabsorption and maldigestion.

5.2. Physical examinations

Physical examination is important and provide important clue into the diagnosis of chronic diarrhoea [45]. Recent weight loss and lymphadenopathy could result from chronic infection or malignancy. Eye finding such as episcleritis or exophthalmia suggests that the diarrhoea is caused by inflammatory bowel disease (IBD) and hyperthyroidism, respectively. The signs that are directly attributed to giardiasis are limited; in fact, there are no specific signs that direct the clinician to suspect giardiasis. However, signs such as anaemia (iron deficiency anaemia), nail pallor, glossitis and koilonychias suggest that there is malabsorption of iron, and cause such as *giardia*, especially in region such as Thailand, should be identified.

5.3. Laboratory diagnosis

Stool microscopy is an important initial test to identify *giardia* trophozoite, blood and faecal leukocyte. Faecal pH test can be done quickly in most centre along with faecal electrolyse to help distinguish secretory diarrhoea from osmotic diarrhoea. A complete blood count, albumin level, erythrocyte sedimentation rate, liver function testing, thyroid-stimulating hormone level and electrolyte levels are important and help exclude other diagnosis such as hyperthyroidism, inflammatory bowel disease, chronic pancreatitis as well as chronic hepatitis [45]. **Figure 2** shows the diagnosis algorithm in managing patients with chronic diarrhoea [45].

6. Conclusion

Giardia is one of the most common water-borne diseases in Thailand and in the world. The finding is particularly more in the area with poor sanitation and unsafe water. In Thailand, the parasites are found in lake and canal but also in water supplies, swimming pool and well. *Giardia* can be transmitted through food and person-person contact. *Giardia* infection usually will be cleared within a few weeks; however, patients might still have intestinal symptoms even after the infection is cleared.

The mechanisms of malabsorption in giardiasis are still obscured. The mechanism such as epithelial dysfunction, villi malformation and immunological disordered has been postulated to be an important cause of malabsorption and maldigestion in giardiasis. It is important to recognise symptoms of chronic giardiasis because this may lead to long-term disability.

Infection with *Giardia* duodenalis may remain asymptomatic or cause acute or chronic diarrhoea. In addition to the intestinal presentation, patient may also develop extra-intestinal complication such as impairment of cognitive function, muscular complications and nutritional deficiencies. Moreover, giardiasis is now recognised as important cause of failure to thrive, stunting and growth retardation in children of the developing countries. In Thailand, giardiasis is considered as public health importance. Although, the long-term consequences of giardiasis is variable, school health program and health education are available for parents and children aimed at reducing the prevalence of parasitic infection and, as a consequence, have a beneficial effect on child growth and development [39].

The diagnosis of giardiasis can be very difficult in asymptomatic individuals. However, the initial steps should include history taking and physical examinations. There are many differential diagnosis of chronic diarrhoea in both adult and children; therefore, good approach in to diagnosis of giardiasis can help reduce hospital health care cost for the patients. Stools sample should be obtained as are sent for microscopy to identify giardia's trophozoite. Serum iron, ferritin, B12 and sign of complications of giardiasis should be investigated.

Treatment aimed directly at clearing the parasite. The antibiotic that is most frequently used is metronidazole. Nutrition supplements, improved health hygiene and sanitation are important aspect into management of giardiasis. Symptoms such as diarrhoea may persist long after the parasites have been cleared.

Author details

Amornnivit Kanokwanvimol

Address all correspondence to: godsmack186@gmail.com

Thammasat University Hospital, Bangkok, Thailand

References

[1] Hisham Nazer.emedicine. Giardiasis [Internet]. 2016. Available from: http://emedicine.medscape.com/article/176718-overview#a3

[2] Caccio SM, Thompson RC, McLauchlin J, Smith HV. Unravelling cryptosporidium giardia epidemiology. Trends in Parasitology. 2005;**21**:430-437

[3] World Health Organization. The World Health Organization report 1998—Life in the 21st Century: A Vision for all. Geneva: World Health Organization Report; 1998. p. 44-45

[4] Cacciò SM, Ryan U. Molecular epidemiology of giardiasis. Molecular and Biochemical Parasitology. 2008;**160**(2):75-80

[5] Dib HH, Lu SQ, Wen SF. Prevalence of *Giardia lamblia* with or without diarrhea in South East, South East Asia and the Far East. Parasitology Research. 2008;**103**:239-251

[6] Al-Mekhlafi MS1, Azlin M, Nor Aini U, Shaik A, Sa'iah A, Fatmah MS, Ismail MG, Ahmad Firdaus MS, Aisah MY, Rozlida AR, Norhayati M. Giardiasis as a predictor

of childhood malnutrition in Orang Asli children in Malaysia. Tropical Medicine and Hygiene. 2005;**9**(99):686-691

[7] Resta-Lenert S, Langford TD, Gillin FD, et al. Altered chlorid secretory responses in HT29/Cl. 19A cells infected with *Giardia lamblia*. Gastroenterology. DOI: 2000118A684. pp. 316-317

[8] Troeger H, Epple H-J, Schneider T, et al. Effect of chronic *Giardia lamblia* infection on epithelial transport and barrier function in human duodenum. Gut. 2007;**56**(3):328-335

[9] Gascon J. Epidemiology, etiology, and pathophysiology of traveler's diarrhea. Digestion. 2006;**73**(Suppl):102-108

[10] Matt Baran-Mickle, The Intestinal Barrier, 2013. Available from: http://robbwolf.com/2013/10/30/impact-nutrition-autoimmune-disease-part-2/

[11] Faubert G. Immune responses to Giardia duodenalis. Clinical Microbiology Reviews. 2000;**13**(1):35-54

[12] Scott KGE, Yu LCH, Buret AG. Role of CD8+ and CD4+ T lymphocytes in jejunal mucosal injury during murine giardiasis. Infection and Immunity. **85**(10):3542

[13] Cevallos A, Carnaby S, James M, et al. Small intestinal injury in a neonatal rat model of giardiasis is strain-dependent. Gastroenterology.

[14] Kaur H, Ghosh S, Samra H, et al. Identification and characterization of an excretory-secretory product from *Giardia lamblia*. Parasitology. 2001;347-356

[15] Jimenez JC, Fontaine J, Grzych JM, et al. Systemic and mucosal responses to oral administration of excretory-secretory antigens from *Giardia* intestinalis. Clinical and Diagnostic Laboratory Immunology. 2004;**11**(1):152-160

[16] Chin AC, Vergnolle N, MacNaughton WK, et al. Proteinase-activated receptor 1 activation induces epithelial apoptosis and increases intestinal permeability. Proceedings of the National Academy of Sciences of the United States of America. 2003;**100**(19):11104-11109

[17] Ankarklev J, Jerlström-Hultqvist J, Ringqvist E, Troell K, Svärd SG. Behind the smile: Cell biology and disease mechanisms of Giardia species. Nature Reviews Microbiology. 2010;**8**:413-422

[18] Mata L. Discussion: Amebiasis, giardiasis, and malnutrition. Reviews of Infectious Diseases. 1982;**4**(4):870. DOI: https://doi.org/10.1093/4.4.870

[19] Roxström-Lindquist K, Palm D, Reiner D, Ringqvist E, Svärd SG. Giardia immunity—An update. Trends in Parasitology. 2006;**22**(1):26-31

[20] Chin AC, Teoh DA, Scott KG, Meddings JB, Macnaughton WK, Buret AG. Strain-dependent induction of enterocyte apoptosis by *Giardia lamblia* disrupts epithelial barrier function in a caspase-3-dependent manner. Infection and Immunity. 2002;**70**(7):3673-3680

[21] Stadelmann B, Merino MC, Persson L, Svärd SG. Arginine consumption by the intestinal parasite *Giardia* intestinalis reduces proliferation of intestinal epithelial. Cell. 2012;

[22] Jonas A, Flanagan PR, Forstner GG. Pathogenesis of mucosal injury in the blind loop syndrome: Brush border enzyme activity and glycoprotein degradation. The Journal of Clinical Investigation. 1977;**60**(6):1321-1330

[23] Kohli A, Bushen OY, Pinkerton RC, Houpt E, Newman RD, Sears CL, Lima AA, Guerrant RL. *Giardia duodenalis* assemblage, clinical presentation and markers of intestinal inflammation in Brazilian children. The American Journal of Tropical Medicine and Hygiene. 2009;**80**(1):16-19

[24] LoGalbo PR, Sampson HA, Buckley RH. Symptomatic giardiasis in three patients with X-linked agammaglobulinemia. The Journal of Pediatrics. 1982;**101**(1):78-80

[25] Levinson JD, Nastro LJ. Giardiasis with total villous atrophy. Gastroenterology. 1978; **74**(2 Pt 1):271-275

[26] Dizdar V, Gilja OH, Hausken T. Increased visceral sensitivity in Giardia-induced postinfectious irritable bowel syndrome and functional dyspepsia. Effect of the 5HT3-antagonist ondansetron. Neurogastroenterology and Motility. 2007;**19**(12):977-982

[27] Rodríguez LA, Ruigómez A. Increased risk of irritable bowel syndrome after bacterial gastroenteritis: Cohort study. BMJ. 1999;**318**(7183):565-566

[28] Spiller RC. Role of infection in irritable bowel syndrome. Journal of Gastroenterology. 2007;**42**(Suppl 17):41-47

[29] Thabane M, Marshall JK. Post-infectious irritable bowel syndrome. World Journal of Gastroenterology. 2009;**15**(29):3591-3596

[30] Barbara G, Stanghellini V, De Giorgio R, Cremon C, Cottrell GS, Santini D, Pasquinelli G, Morselli-Labate AM, Grady EF, Bunnett NW, et al. Activated mast cells in proximity to colonic nerves correlate with abdominal pain in irritable bowel syndrome. Gastroenterology. 2004;**126**(3):693-702

[31] Simsek Z, Zeyrek FY, Kurcer MA. Effect of Giardia infection on growth and psychomotor development of children aged 0-5 years. Journal of Tropical Pediatrics. 2004;**50**:90-93

[32] Guerrant DI, Moore SR, Lima AA, Patrick PD, Schorling JB, Guerrant RL. Association of early childhood diarrhea and cryptosporidiosis with impaired physical fitness and cognitive function four-seven years later in a poor urban community in northeast Brazil. The American Journal of Tropical Medicine and Hygiene. 1999;**61**(5):707-701

[33] Thompson RC, Reynoldson JA, Mendis AH. Giardia and giardiasis. Advances in Parasitology. 1993;**32**:71-160

[34] Bergman P, Graham J. An approach to "failure to thrive". Australian Family Physician. 2005;**34**:725-729

[35] Farthing MJ, Mata L, Urrutia JJ, Kronmal RA. Natural history of Giardia infection of infants and children in rural Guatemala and its impact on physical growth. The American Journal of Clinical Nutrition. 1986;**43**:395-405

[36] Mitchell CM, Bradford CM, Kapur U. *Giardia lamblia* trophozoites in an ultrasound-guided fine-needle aspiration of a pancreatic mucinous neoplasm. Diagnostic Cytopathology. 2011;**39**:352-353

[37] Kurita A, Maguchi H, Takahashi K, Katanuma A, Osanai M, Kin T, Yane K, Hashigo S, Ohtsubo M. Small pancreatic cancer with giardiasis: A case report. Pancreas. 2010;**39**:943-945

[38] Ajjampur SS, Koshy B, Venkataramani M, Sarkar R, Joseph AA, Jacob KS, Ward H, Kang G. Effect of cryptosporidial and giardial diarrhoea on social maturity, intelligence and physical growth in children in a semi-urban slum in south India. Annals of Tropical Paediatrics. 2011;**31**:205-212

[39] Berkman DS, Lescano AG, Gilman RH, Lopez SL, Black MM. Effects of stunting, diarrhoeal disease, and parasitic infection during infancy on cognition in late childhood: A follow-up study. Lancet. 2002;**359**:564-571

[40] Niehaus MD, Moore SR, Patrick PD, Derr LL, Lorntz B, Lima AA, Guerrant RL. Early childhood diarrhea is associated with diminished cognitive function 4 to 7 years later in children in a northeast Brazilian shantytown. The American Journal of Tropical Medicine and Hygiene. 2002;**66**:590-593

[41] Celiksöz A, Aciöz M, Değerli S, Cinar Z, Elaldi N, Erandaç M. Effects of giardiasis on school success, weight and height indices of primary school children in Turkey. Pediatrics International. 2005;**47**:567-571

[42] de Deungria M, Rao R, Wobken JD, Luciana M, Nelson CA, Georgieff MK. Perinatal iron deficiency decreases cytochrome c oxidase (CytOx) activity in selected regions of neonatal rat brain. Pediatric Research. 2000;**48**(2):169-176

[43] Veenemans J, Schouten LR, Ottenhof MJ, Mank TG, Uges DR, Mbugi EV, Demir AY, Kraaijenhagen RJ, Savelkoul HF, Verhoef H. Effect of preventive supplementation with zinc and other micronutrients on non-malarial morbidity in Tanzanian pre-school children: A randomized trial. PloS One. 2012;

[44] Genovese A, Spadaro G, Santoro L, Gasparo Rippa P, Onorati AM, Marone G. Giardiasis as a cause of hypokalemic myopathy in congenital immunodeficiency. International Journal of Clinical & Laboratory Research. 1996;**26**(2):132-135

[45] Juckett G, Trivedi R. West Virginia University, Morgantown, West VirginiaEvaluation of chronic diarrhoea [Internet]. American Family Physician. 2011;**84**(10):1119-1126

Chapter 4

Giardiasis: Livestock and Companion Animals

Joyce Siwila

Additional information is available at the end of the chapter

http://dx.doi.org/10.5772/intechopen.70874

Abstract

Giardia spp. are flagellates that are found in the intestinal tract of humans and domestic and wildlife animals, including birds and amphibians, worldwide. The genus *Giardia* comprises several species which are morphologically similar. *Giardia* infections have been reported widely in livestock and companion animals with varying prevalence in different parts of the world. Giardiasis, the disease cause by *Giardia*, may result in numerous episodes of diarrhoea, especially in young animals, which in turn adversely affect production resulting in economic loses. The affected animals may also act as a source of zoonotic infections. Evidence of infection in both animals and humans of *Giardia duodenalis* especially of assemblage A and B has firmly established giardiasis as a zoonotic disease. The zoonotic assemblage A and B have been reported in livestock (cattle, sheep, goats, pigs) and companion animals (dogs, cats, horses). However, questions regarding the direct transmission of *Giardia* from domestic animals to humans still need to be explored. Appropriate prevention and control measures are cardinal in preventing both animal and human infections. This chapter discusses *G. duodenalis* infection and the disease including treatment options in livestock and companion animals.

Keywords: *Giardia, Giardia duodenalis*, giardiasis, livestock, companion animals, treatment

1. Introduction

For years, man has relied on livestock for food, drought power, hides and other production activities. In less developed countries, livestock production is mostly done using traditional methods due to limited resources and these small-scale production systems accounts for most agricultural output in these countries [1]. On the other hand, companion animals are equally kept throughout the world. Dogs and cats are particularly kept as pets with increasing numbers in nations that previously did not do so but kept dogs mostly for security. Now, dogs are widely used for different purposes, including companionship, life-saving actions, security as well as hunting and farming [2, 3]. Other than entertainment and sports, horses are also being kept for companionship. These livestock and companion animals are however hosts to many parasites, some of which have detrimental effects on the health and productivity of those affected. Protozoa such as *Giardia duodenalis* affect a wide range of domestic and wild animals, with serious clinical consequences especially in young animals.

G. duodenalis (syn. *Giardia lamblia, Giardia intestinalis*), a flagellate protozoan parasite, and the aetiological agent of giardiasis, is one of the most prevalent and widespread intestinal parasite in humans and several vertebrate animal species worldwide [4]. The taxonomy of the genus is mainly based on morphology and genetic evidence. According to these criteria, six species have been recognised in the genus *Giardia* and these include *G. duodenalis* in humans and other mammals, *G. agilis* in amphibians, *G. muris* and *G. microti* in rodents, *G. psittaci* and *G. ardeae* in birds. In recent years, phylogenetic analysis and enzyme electrophoresis have revealed the existence of eight assemblages A–H within the species *G. duodenalis* [5–7]. *Giardia* from humans appears to fall exclusively into Assemblage A and B while C and D are dog specific assemblages. Assemblage E is isolated from hooved animals, a characteristic of isolates from sheep, goats, cattle and pigs [8]. Cats are hosts F or Assemblage F while rats are hosts for Assemblage G [9, 10]. Assemblage H has been reported in the grey seal [11].

G. duodenalis is a frequently encountered intestinal parasite of domestic animals, especially livestock, dogs and cats. *Giardia* infections have been reported widely in livestock and companion animals with varying prevalence in different parts of the world, but high frequency was mostly in dairy calves [12–16]. As a parasite, *Giardia* has a broad host range, however, the adverse consequences of infection and its pathogenic potential are best recognised in humans [6]. It causes an estimated 2.8×10^8 human cases per annum [17]. In Asia, Africa and Latin America, about 200 million people have symptomatic giardiasis with some 500,000 new cases reported each year [18]. Its simple life cycle involving an environmentally resistant cyst (**Figure 1**) provides greater opportunities for the parasite to be transmitted directly from one infected individual to another, or indirectly through contamination of the environment or food [4].

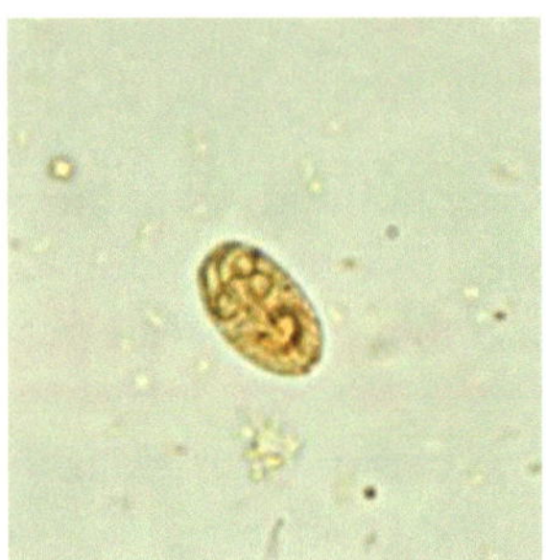

Figure 1. *Giardia* cyst: wet smear stained with iodine (source: https://www.cdc.gov/dpdx/giardiasis/index.html).

2. Transmission and clinical disease

The cyst is the infective stage and represents the resting stage of the organism. Its rigid outer wall protects the parasite against changes in environmental temperature, dehydration and chlorination, all of which would destroy the trophozoite [6, 19, 20] . Transmission occurs by the faecal-oral route, either by direct contact with an infected host, or through contaminated food or water [21, 22]. Mechanical transmission of the parasite through insect vectors has also been reported [23]. Factors that facilitate infection include overcrowding, the high excretion of cysts by infected animals and the low infectious dose (between 10 and 25 cysts) [24, 25].

Giardia is not invasive and therefore lives and multiplies by asexual multiplication on the luminal surface of the small intestine of the vertebrate host [6]. Although the pathogenesis of *Giardia* is not completely understood, the pathophysiological process is initiated by infection with the parasite resulting in variable clinical signs such as abdominal pain, diarrhoea and weight loss [26]. A rise in numbers of intraepithelial lymphocytes increases epithelial permeability. Activation of T-lymphocytes has also been observed in *Giardia* infections [27, 28]. Trophozoite toxins and T-cell activation initiate a diffuse shortening of brush border microvilli and decreased activity of the small intestinal brush border enzymes, particularly lipase, proteases and disaccharidases [29–31]. The microvillus shortening leads to a decrease in overall absorptive area in the small intestine and an impaired uptake of water, electrolytes and nutrients resulting in malabsorptive diarrhoea [29, 32]. The steatorrhoea and mucous diarrhoea usually observed in giardiasis are attributed to reduced activity of lipase and increased production of mucin by goblet cells [33]. Severity of the disease is dependent on factors like developmental, nutritional and immunity of the host as well as virulence factors of the parasite [30, 34, 35]. Although gross intestinal lesions are rarely observed, microscopic lesions consisting of villous atrophy and cuboidal enterocytes may be reported [33].

3. Giardiasis in livestock

3.1. Cattle

In cattle, *Giardia* is considered an important emerging parasite of dairy cattle and also as a cause of zoonotic disease with negative effect on public health [19]. Calves have been reported to be infected with *G. duodenalis* as early as 4 days of age, and the highest intensity of cyst excretion of 10^5–10^6 cysts per gram of faeces between the ages of 1 and 3 months has been documented [36, 37]. A periparturient rise in cyst excretion has also been demonstrated [37]. Transmission occurs among infected calves as well as chronically infected adults [12, 38, 39] and is particularly high among dairy calves [38, 39]. There are four main proposed cycles of transmission that are believed to maintain host-specific and zoonotic assemblages of *Giardia* in mammalian hosts: human cycle, livestock cycle, dog/cat cycle and wildlife cycle (**Figure 2**).

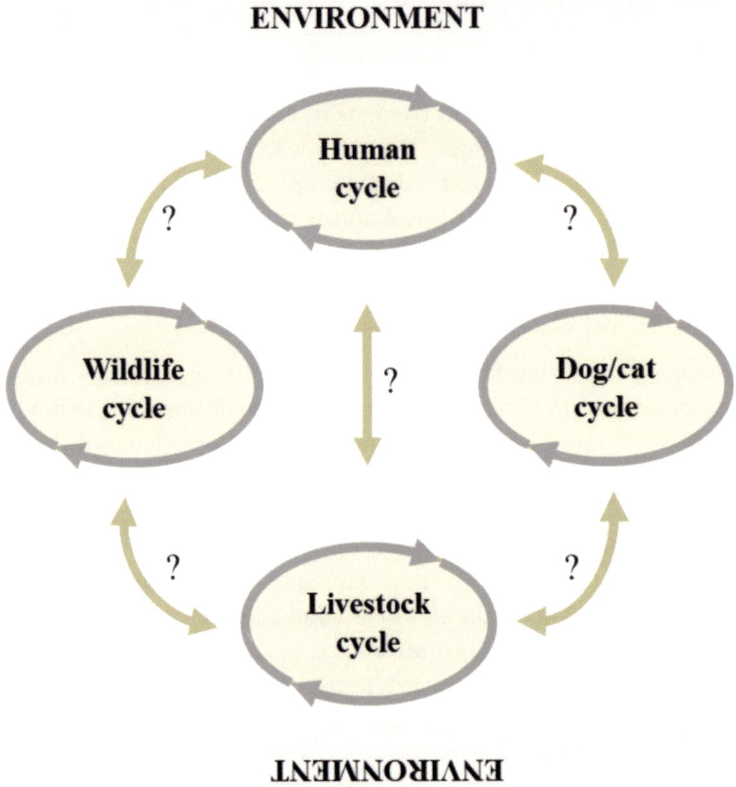

Figure 2. Transmission cycles of *Giardia duodenalis* (*frequency of transmission is unknown*).

The livestock cycle is thought to maintain Assemblage E within the livestock group [6, 40, 41]. The other cycles maintain the assemblages in the specific hosts. For example, assemblages A and B can be maintained by direct transmission between humans, assemblage C and D between dogs (e.g. puppies in a breeding kennel) and wildlife genotypes among various wildlife species. Some assemblages, however, infect other animal species and humans. The frequency of transmission is however not very clear and still under debate. Zoonotic species have been reported in wildlife, but their role as a potentials reservoir for human infection still requires further molecular epidemiological research [4].

The resultant giardiasis from *G. duodenalis* infection can result in diarrhoea that does not respond to treatment with antibiotic or anti-coccidia drugs [33, 36, 42]. *Giardia* has been implicated as an aetiological agent alone and in combination with other enteric pathogens in calf diarrhoea [36, 38, 43, 44]. Infection may also result in numerous diarrhoea episodes which in turn adversely affects production and result in economic loses for farmers [45]. In younger calves, especially below 6 months of age, the excretion of watery faeces with a mucoid appearance may be the only indication of infection with the parasite. Chronic cases of giardiasis in calves may impact negatively on performance which may be reflected in reduced weight gain, impaired feed efficiency and decreased carcass weight. This was demonstrated in experimentally infected lambs [43].

Giardia has been found in both beef and dairy cattle throughout the world with varying prevalence. Infection rates can be as high as 100% [36–38, 46–50]. The infection pattern of *Giardia* appears similar between beef and dairy cattle [36, 37] with cysts appearing in the faeces at approximately 4 weeks of age [12, 36, 38] . Both dairy and beef calves may harbour more than one genotype of *G. duodenalis*, which can be of zoonotic significance [12, 51, 52]. Assemblages A, B and E have been detected in cattle; Assemblages A and B also infect humans [53, 54]. As calves infected with *Giardia* shed large numbers of cysts, there is concern that cattle could represent a reservoir of *G. duodenalis* with the potential to cause disease in humans either through direct contact or by contamination of food and/or water supplies [36]. Because of the risk of contamination of water supplies by water borne parasites such as *Giardia*, it is normally recommended that animal facilities should be located away from streams, lakes, dams and rivers whenever possible, and waterways should be fenced-off in pasture lands in order to prevent possible run-off into these water sources [55].

3.2. Sheep

The prevalence of *G. duodenalis* infection in sheep varies considerably and may be as high as 38% in adult sheep and 68% in lambs [56–60]. In a study in central China [61], the prevalence of *G. duodenalis* was 12.36% in pre-weaned lambs and 5.74% in post-weaned sheep [61]. Other studies have also reported great variability in *Giardia* prevalence: in Canada, prevalence of giardiasis was higher in lambs (57%) than in adults (9%) [62]; in Brazil, lambs had a 32% infection rate while that for ewes was 2%; [63]; and in Mongolia, China, lambs had a significantly higher infection rate than ewes (8.6 versus 0.9%, respectively) [64]. All the findings from these studies suggest that the infection rates of *Giardia* tend to decline as the age of the animals increases. However, the opposite has also been reported. In some studies in Australia, a much higher prevalence of was detected in post-weaned lambs and sheep (44%) than in pre-weaned sheep (11.1%) [56, 65]. In a study in Maryland, USA, the prevalence of giardiasis was higher in post-parturient ewes (12%) than in lambs (4%) [59]. Host age and immune status of the host affect the severity of the disease [6] but other factors such as the number of specimens examined, the age structure of the herds, management procedures and the health status of the animals may account for the discrepancies or variations in the infection rates in the different populations [61].

Because of the unexpectedly high levels of infection in sheep, sheep have long been considered a reservoir of human infections [56, 61, 66–68]. In most cases, infections are asymptomatic but infected animals are carriers shedding large numbers of cysts into the environment [58]. Even if most infections are asymptomatic, infections in lambs may result in a malabsorption syndrome, decreased feed efficiency and subsequently a decreased weight gain and sometimes death [19, 43, 69]. In the study by [69], excretion of malodorous and poorly formed faeces was observed. Furthermore, giardiasis may have a negative effect on time to slaughter of the sheep [19, 43] therefore, negatively affecting producers' income.

Three assemblages of *G. duodenalis* have been recognised in sheep, livestock assemblage E, and the two zoonotic assemblages A and B [13, 56, 59]. The non-zoonotic assemblage E is the most frequently reported compared to the zoonotic ones [59, 66, 68, 69]. However, assemblage E appears to occur most frequently in cattle compared to other livestock; this was demonstrated by an extensive, longitudinal study of dairy herds in Australia over several months and another study in Canada [12, 56, 70].

3.3. Goats

In small ruminants, there are considerably more surveys from sheep populations than goat populations and therefore fewer publications on *Giardia* in goats. Furthermore, only a few molecular studies regarding *Giardia* have been performed worldwide [13, 58, 71–74] compared to other ruminant hosts (see [4]). In the reported studies, *Giardia* prevalence was reported to range from <10 to >40% depending on the age, geographical location and diagnostic technique used [75]. Infections are normally significantly higher in pre-weaned goat kids compared to that in older goat kids [74]. Most infections are asymptomatic, however, foul-smelling diarrhoea which is lightly coloured, greasy and mixed with mucous; reduced weight gain are clinical signs that may be observed, mostly in young animals that are symptomatic [71]. A study in Spain reported a high infection rate in young animals, agreeing with the hypothesis that to a great extent, young animals contribute to the environmental contamination with *Giardia* cysts [71]. A study in Nigeria also reported a high prevalence (46.9%) in goats with pre-weaned (≤3 months) goats having a much higher prevalence (58.1%) compared to those that were over 3 months (38.2%) [74].

Even though a large number of *G. duodenalis* genotyping studies in ruminants report a higher occurrence of genotype E, with genotypes A and B being less frequent [13, 58, 76, 77], other studies, [13, 72] have reported zoonotic genotype A infections in goats in Belgium and Côte d'Ivoire, respectively. In Malaysia, one study [73] reported genotypes A and B in goats. These findings suggest that goats could be a potential source of zoonotic infection.

3.4. Pigs

There is limited information on the *Giardia* infections in pigs. From the limited studies, *Giardia* infections have been reported in all age groups from nursing piglets to boars and sows worldwide, from Australia, Asia, Europe and North America, Africa with varying prevalence ranging between 0.1 and 20% [62, 78–86]. Natural infections are typically asymptomatic with no evidence of illness.

Both assemblages E and A have been identified in pigs with assemblage E being most common [4]. In one study in Australia, assemblage E was the most common genotype detected in positive specimens of both pre-weaned (64%) and post-weaned (67%) pigs [87]. In Denmark, assemblage E was also the most common genotype, being identified in 62% of samples from post-weaned pigs, while assemblage A was detected in only 12% of specimens [85]. Interestingly, the canine assemblage D has also been reported in pigs [85, 88].

Since pigs also harbour the zoonotic assemblage A, they should be considered as potential sources of infection. One case–control study in eastern England found an association between giardiasis and exposure to farm animals, pigs included [89].

4. Companion animals

4.1. Dogs and cats

Giardia is commonly recovered from the faeces of both symptomatic and asymptomatic dogs worldwide [90, 91]. Several studies have reported high prevalence of *Giardia* in stool samples of companion animals (i.e. cats and dogs) (reviewed by [92]). *Giardia* infection rates in dogs differ considerably based on many variables, including the composition of dog populations (owned/stray/kennel), the test used for diagnosis and its sensitivity. Similar to other animal species, severity of disease depends on host age and ability of the immunity to eliminate the infection. Reports of giardiasis range from 0.1% in owned dogs to as high as 100% in kenneled dogs, the risk factor being overcrowding and intensive contact between large numbers of dogs sharing the same shelter in kenneled dogs. This favours transmission of infections [6, 15, 93–96]. Some studies have indicated *Giardia* to be the most common enteric parasite of dogs and cats. For example, studies in Australia found that *G. duodenalis* was the most common enteric parasite of domestic dogs and cats [97, 98] while [99] also reported the parasite to be widely prevalent in dogs and cats in the USA. The prevalence of *Giardia* in these companion animals is however, believed to be underestimated because of the following reasons: the low sensitivity of the conventional detection methods, cyst excretion is intermittent and the disease is usually subclinical [98].

In most of the studies that have been conducted in dogs, puppies, free-roaming dogs, and shelter dogs have been shown to be at higher risk for infection than adult dogs and owned dogs [15, 94]. Transmission of the parasite appears to be maintained within the dog/cat cycle (**Figure 2**) as evidenced from the host specific assemblage C/D and F commonly isolated in dogs and cats respectively [15, 100]. However, zoonotic transmission of *Giardia* between humans and dogs in the same household has been reported previously [101]. In another study in Brazil, zoonotic assemblage A1 was isolated from dogs and children in the same locality suggesting the existence of a zoonotic cycle of the parasite in that community [102], and a study in Thailand revealed that dogs were a potential source of *Giardia* infections for humans [103]. In this study [103], assemblages A (79%) and B (21%) in addition to the dog specific assemblages C (12%) and D (31%) were isolated from the 104 dogs tested. In the United States, one study reported that 28 and 41% of client-owned dogs presenting with infection with *Giardia* to veterinary clinics had potentially zoonotic assemblages A and B, respectively, while 15 and 16% had host specific assemblages C and D, respectively [104]. The findings from the American study suggest the possibility of the potential for transmission of non-canine-specific assemblages from owners to their dogs as well as zoonotic transmission from dogs to humans. Furthermore, such reports highlight the possibility of two transmission cycles existing in domestic urban environments, that is, transmission of dog-specific assemblages among dogs and the possible transmission of assemblage A between pets and humans. However, it has been reported that in household dogs, the frequency of dog-to-dog transmission may be lower because they are less crowded than kenneled dogs where prevalence is normally higher due to intensive contact among a large number of dogs [54, 91].

Although *Giardia* is common in dogs and cats, it is rarely associated with clinical disease and affected animals suffer minimal consequences of the disease, but may act as a source of zoonotic infection [103, 104]. However, complications such as persistent infections and impairment of growth and development may occur especially in young animals such as puppies and kittens [105]. Such infections with manifestation of clinical signs are usually associated with kennel or cattery setup, where there is overcrowding [106].

4.2. Horses

There is very few data on *Giardia* in horses and giardiasis is an uncommon condition in these animals. However, the parasite may be commonly found in faeces of asymptomatic animals. The parasite was first reported in horses in South Africa in 1921 [107]. Since then a number of reports have been made regarding the presence of the parasite in horses of all age groups. Relatively high rates of giardiasis among foals (17–35%) and lactating mares (1.9–27.8%) have been documented using the fluorescent antibody method [38]. Lower rates have been observed in weanlings (0–9.1%) [108]. Varying prevalence of giardiasis has been reported in different geographic areas and they differ considerably between locations [62, 109, 110] with age and physiological status of the animal playing an important role in the infection rates [38, 110].

Although giardiasis in horses has been found to be associated with diarrhoea, poor hair coat, ill thrift and weight loss [111, 112], infected horses rarely show any clinical signs [108] and no subclinical consequences have been reported previously. However, infected horses may show signs ranging from a mild and self-limiting to, occasionally, severe diarrhoea (with heavy infections). These are commonly seen in young and aged or immunologically suppressed horses [110, 113, 114]. However, some studies have reported no shedding of *Giardia* cysts in young and older horses [115].

G. duodenalis assemblages A, B, and E have been detected in horses [110, 116]. A study in Italy also confirmed the presence of both animal and human sub-assemblage of *G. duodenalis* in horses [117]. However, assemblage E appears to be more common in these animals [110]. Because assemblages A and B are known to infect humans [6, 118], horses could represent a reservoir of *G. duodenalis* with the potential to cause disease in humans through direct contact or by contamination of food and/or water supplies.

5. Diagnosis

The diagnosis of giardiasis is commonly established by microscopic identification of cysts or less commonly trophozoites in faecal specimens stained with trichrome (**Figure 3**) or iron

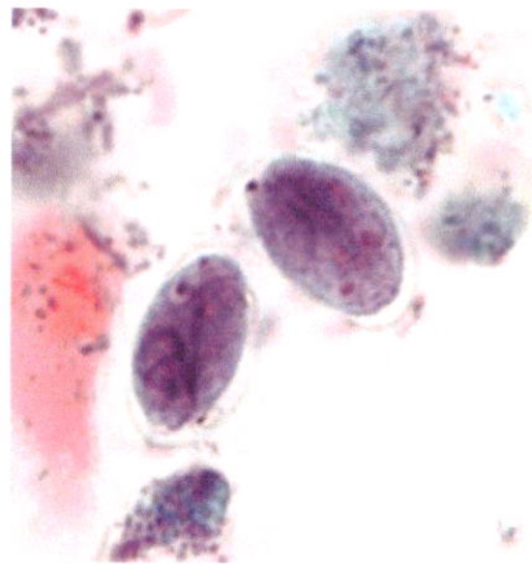

Figure 3. *Giardia* cysts stained with trichrome stain (source: https://www.cdc.gov/dpdx/giardiasis/index.html).

haematoxylin. This follows the application of faecal concentration techniques, especially zinc sulphate flotation and centrifugation [119]. Direct smear or wet mount examination for trophozoites can also be performed. However, because of the cyclical nature of cyst excretion, several samples need to be examined to detect the organism [120]. The disadvantage of microscopy is that it is of limited epidemiological value as it does not indicate the source of the infection [6].

Faecal immunoassays have been developed and these have improved the sensitivity of detecting the parasite in faecal specimens. The sensitivity and specificity of different assays is reported to range from 87 to 100% [121, 122]. Enzyme-linked immunosorbent assay (ELISA) is the mostly used immunoassay and it has enhanced the detection of the parasite in field samples and a number of kits are commercially available [120]. Furthermore, the development of direct immunofluorescence microscopy (antigen detection) has generally improved the sensitivity of detecting and quantifying faecal *Giardia* cysts and may allow for more accurate determination of prevalence rates and cyst excretion intensities compared to the conventional microscopy [46]. However, despite antigen detection being more sensitive than conventional microscopy, the method cannot discriminate between species or morphologically similar organisms. The other disadvantage is the need for a fluorescent microscope which is costly [123].

To overcome the non-discriminatory nature of the conventional microscopy, molecular techniques, particularly PCR-based procedures have been developed and have greater sensitivity and specificity than the techniques that rely on microscopy and/or immunodiagnosis [98]. For example, in a survey of dogs in India, microscopy detected only 3% prevalence compared to 20% with PCR [101]. The molecular methods are also able to provide information on the genotypes and species of *Giardia*, information that is necessary for determining the source of infection. PCR, when combined with restriction fragment length polymorphism (RFLP) analysis is faster when compared to sequencing which is also costly [124]. Although PCR has high sensitivity, results may be affected by amplification inhibitors and barriers to DNA extraction in faecal samples [125]. Moreover, PCR assays are very costly for diagnostic laboratory use [126] and are therefore commonly used in research.

Serodiagnosis cannot be used to differentiate between present and previous infection and is therefore not useful for the diagnosis of giardiasis.

6. Treatment

Treatment of giardiasis in livestock is through use of fenbendazole and albendazole, which have been shown to be effective in the elimination of *Giardia* from both housed and range calves [32, 127–129] as well as improving the mucosal microvillus structure and function within a week [129]. In sheep, treatment with fenbendazole at a dose of 10 mg/kg for three consecutive days, has been shown to successfully clear the infection. In an outbreak of giardiasis on a sheep farm, *Giardia*-infected lambs (30–90 days of age) presenting with malabsorption, decreased weight gain, and reduced feed efficiency recovered rapidly from the symptoms and poor weight gain after treatment with fenbendazole [69]. Similarly, in calves experimentally infected with *G. duodenalis* and treated with fenbendazole, a significant difference in weight gain was noticed between fenbendazole-treated and untreated calves. Animals in the treatment group gained on average 2.86 kg (equal to 102 g per day) more than the animals in the control group [27]. However, in some other treatment studies where fenbendazole or paromomycin sulphate were used, differences in mean body weight, average daily weight gain, or feed intake between the control and treated groups were not significant, although there was a slightly higher weight gain and lower occurrence of diarrhoea in the treated groups [12, 42].

In dogs and cats, fenbendazole is the commonly used therapy, normally given once daily for 3–5 days. Albendazole can be used but it has been associated with bone marrow suppression in both dogs and cats, and so no longer being used in both animal species [130]. Vaccines for *Giardia* in dogs and cats have been developed and they are reported to have the ability to reduce the duration of shedding of cysts which may subsequently reduce environmental contamination [131]. A prolonged treatment up to 5 days was shown not to be statistically better than treatment for three consecutive days [132]. On the other hand, metronidazole has been used to treat giardiasis in horses, with resolution of clinical signs after treatment [112].

7. Conclusions

Giardia infections are prevalent in livestock and companion animals. A number of studies have reported and genotyped *Giardia* in domestic animals, particularly livestock and companion animals, and have found that they may be infected with zoonotic or species-specific genotypes. However, there is still limited information on infection rates in pigs and horses. Further, the role of these animals and dogs in the zoonotic transmission of *Giardia* still needs further investigation. Studies reporting the existence of zoonotic assemblages in both animals and humans in the same locality (e.g. for dogs) emphasise the need for further studies on zoonotic transmission of *Giardia*. Such information will assist in further highlighting the public health significance of *Giardia*. Increased interaction and the nature of the interaction between companion animals and their owners can determine whether zoonotic infection occurs or not.

Economic implications of the disease in terms of treatment costs that the farmers have to incur cannot be overlooked especially in livestock (particularly dairy calves). Giardiasis adversely affects production; and chronic cases may impact negatively on the performance of affected animals resulting in reduced weight gain, impaired feed efficiency and delayed maturity. These loses translate into food loses.

Unfortunately, giardiasis in humans is not a health priority in most countries but the effect of the parasite in terms of patient well-being and its effect on quality of life have been highlighted by many authors, highlighting its impact on human health.

A better understanding of the disease in animals (livestock and companion animals), the species and transmission patterns is necessary for appropriate prevention and control strategies which should result in increased livestock production and reduced treatment costs for the farmers or animal owners. More molecular epidemiological studies are required especially in areas where these have not been conducted such as sub-Saharan Africa to understand and probably be able to relate human and animal infections. Treatment of *Giardia* infection in both livestock and companion animals is recommended whether or not they are clinically ill, because of the potential for zoonotic transmission.

Author details

Joyce Siwila

Address all correspondence to: siwilaj@yahoo.co.uk

Department of Clinical Studies, University of Zambia School of Veterinary Medicine, Lusaka, Zambia

References

[1] FAO. Major Livestock Production Systems in Africa. Available from: http://www.fao.org/wairdocs/ilri/x5547e/x5547e0o.htm. [Accessed: 3 April 2017]

[2] Beck AM. The impact of the canine cleanup law: Both dogs and people profit. Environment: Science and Policy for Sustainable Development. 1979;**21**:197. DOI: 10.1080/00139157.1979.9931200

[3] Szabova E, Juris P, Miterpakova M, Antolova D, Papajova I, Sefcikova H. Prevalence of important zoonotic parasites in dog populations from the Slovak Republic. Helminthologia. 2007;**44**:170-176. DOI: 10.2478/s11687-007-0027-3

[4] Feng Y, Xiao L. Zoonotic potential and molecular epidemiology of *Giardia* species and giardiasis. Clinical Microbiology Reviews. 2011;**24**:110-140. DOI: 10.1128/CMR.00033-10

[5] Berrilli F, Di Cave D, De Liberato C, Franco A, Scaramozzino P, Orecchia P. Genotype characterisation of *Giardia duodenalis* isolates from domestic and farm animals by SSU-rRNA gene sequencing. Veterinary Parasitology. 2004;**122**:193-199. DOI: 10.1016/j.vetpar.2004.04.008

[6] Thompson RCA. The zoonotic significance and molecular epidemiology of *Giardia* and giardiasis. Veterinary Parasitology. 2004;**126**:15-35. DOI: 10.1016/j.vetpar.2004.09.008

[7] Heyworth MF. *Giardia duodenalis* genetic assemblages and hosts. Parasite. 2016;**23**:13. DOI: 10.1051/parasite/2016013

[8] Ey PL, Mansouri M, Kulda J, Nohýnková E, Monis PT, Andrews RH, Mayrhofer G. Genetic analysis of *Giardia* from hoofed farm animals reveals artiodactyl-specific and potentially zoonotic genotypes. Journal of Eukaryotic Microbiology. 1997;**44**:626-635. DOI: 10.1111/j.1550-7408.1997.tb05970.x

[9] Hopkins RM, Meloni BP, Groth DM, Wetherall JD, Reynoldson JA, Thompson RCA, Ribososomal RNA. sequencing reveals differences between the genotypes of *Giardia* isolates recovered from humans and dogs in the same locality. Journal of Parasitology. 1997;**83**:44. DOI: 10.2307/3284315

[10] Bowman DD. Georgis' Parasitology for Veterinarians. 9th ed. Saunders Elsevier. St Louis Missouri. 2009; ISBN: 978-1-4160-4412-3

[11] Lasek-Nesselquist E, Welch DM, Sogin ML. The identification of a new *Giardia duodenalis* assemblage in marine vertebrates and a preliminary analysis of *G. duodenalis* population biology in marine systems. International Journal for Parasitology. 2010;**40**:1063-1074. DOI: 10.1016/j.ijpara.2010.02.015

[12] O'Handley R, Olson M, Fraser D, Adams P, Thompson R. Prevalence and genotypic characterization of *Giardia* in dairy calves from Western Australia and Western Canada. Veterinary Parasitology. 2000;**90**:193-200. DOI: http://dx.doi.org/10.1016/S0304-4017(00)00235-1

[13] Geurden T, Geldhof P, Levecke B, Martens C, Berkvens D, Casaert S, Vercruysse J, Claerebout E. Mixed *Giardia duodenalis* assemblage A and E infections in calves. International Journal for Parasitology. 2008;**38**:259-264. DOI: 10.1016/j.ijpara.2007.07.016

[14] Lebbad M, Mattsson J, Christensson D, Ljungstrom B, Backhans A, Andersson J, Svard S. From mouse to moose: Multilocus genotyping of *Giardia* isolates from various animal species. Veterinary Parasitology. 2010;**168**:231-239. DOI: 10.1016/j.vetpar.2009.11.003

[15] Mircean V, Györke A, Cozma V. Prevalence and risk factors of *Giardia duodenalis* in dogs in Romania. Veterinary Parasitology. 2012;**184**:325-329. DOI: 10.1016/j.vetpar.2011.08.022

[16] Minetti C, Taweenan W, Hogg R, Featherstone C, Randle N, Latham SM, Wastling JM. Occurrence and diversity of *Giardia duodenalis* assemblages in livestock in the UK. Transboundary and Emerging Diseases. 2013;**61**:e60-e67. DOI: 10.1111/tbed.12075

[17] Lane S, Lloyd D. Current trends in research into the waterborne parasite *Giardia*. Critical Reviews in Microbiology. 2002;**28**:123-147. DOI: 10.1080/1040-840291046713

[18] WHO. The World Health Report 1996. Fighting Disease Fostering Development. Geneva: World Health Organization; 1996

[19] Olson M, O'Handley R, Ralston B, McAllister T, Thompson R. Update on *Cryptosporidium* and *Giardia* infections in cattle. Trends in Parasitology. 2004;**20**:151-198. DOI: 10.1016/j.pt.2004.01.015

[20] Thompson R, Monis P. *Giardia* – from genome to proteome. Advances in Parasitology. 2012;**78**:57-95. DOI: http://dx.doi.org/10.1016/B978-0-12-394303-3.00003-7

[21] Gow S, Waldner C. An examination of the prevalence of and risk factors for shedding of *Cryptosporidium* spp. and *Giardia* spp. in cows and calves from western Canadian cow-calf herds. Veterinary Parasitology. 2006;**137**:50-61. DOI: 10.1016/j.vetpar.2005.05.071

[22] Hamnes I, Gjerde B, Robertson L. Prevalence of *Giardia* and *Cryptosporidium* in dairy calves in three areas of Norway. Veterinary Parasitology, 2006;**140**:204-216. DOI: http://dx.doi.org/10.1016/j.vetpar.2006.03.024

[23] Graczyk TK, Grimes BH, Knight R, Da Silva AJ, Pieniazek NJ, Veal DA. Detection of *Cryptosporidium* parvum and *Giardia lamblia* carried by synanthropic flies by combined fluorescent in situ hybridization and a monoclonal antibody. American Journal of Tropical Medicine and Hygiene. 2003;**68**:228-232. DOI: https://doi.org/10.4269/ajtmh.2003.68.228

[24] Rendtorff RC. The experimental transmission of human intestinal protozoan parasites. II. *Giardia lamblia* cysts given in capsules. American Journal of Hygiene. 1954;**59**:209-220. PMID: 13138586 ISSN: 0096-5294

[25] Faubert GM. The immune response to *Giardia*. Parasitology Today. 1996;**12**:140-145. DOI: https://doi.org/10.1016/0169-4758(96)10004-1

[26] Buret AG. Pathophysiology of enteric infections with *Giardia duodenalis*. Parasite. 2008;**15**:261-265. DOI: https://doi.org/10.1051/parasite/2008153261

[27] Geurden T, Vandenhoute E, Pohle H, Casaert S, De Wilde N, Vercruysse J, Claerebout E. The effect of a fenbendazole treatment on cyst excretion and weight gain in calves experimentally infected with *Giardia duodenalis*. Veterinary Parasitology. 2010;**169**:18-23. DOI: http://dx.doi.org/10.1016/j.vetpar.2009.12.027

[28] Koh W, Geurden T, Paget T, O'Handley R, Steuart R, Thompson R, Buret A. *Giardia duodenalis* assemblage-specific induction of apoptosis and tight junction disruption in human intestinal epithelial cells: Effects of mixed infections. Journal of Parasitology. 2013;**99**:353-358. doi: http://dx.doi.org/10.1645/GE-3021.1

[29] McDonnell P, Scott K, Teoh D, Olson M, Upcroft J, Upcroft P, Buret A. *Giardia duodenalis* trophozoites isolated from a parrot (Cacatua galerita) colonize the intestinal tracts of domestic kittens and lambs. Veterinary Parasitology. 2002;**111**:31-46. DOI: http://dx.doi.org/10.1016/S0304-4017(02)00349-7

[30] Scott KG, Meddings JB, Kirk DR, Lees-Miller SP, Buret AG. Intestinal infection with *Giardia* spp. reduces epithelial barrier function in a myosin light chain kinase-dependent fashion. Gastroenterology 2002;**123**:1179-1190. DOI: http://dx.doi.org/10.1053/gast.2002.36002

[31] Buret AG. Mechanisms of epithelial dysfunction in giardiasis. Gut 2007;**56**:328-335. DOI: http://dx.doi.org/10.1136/gut.2006.107771

[32] O'Handley M, Buret A, McAllister T, Jelinski M, Olson M. Giardiasis in dairy calves: effects of fenbendazole treatment on intestinal structure and function. International Journal for Parasitology 2001;**31**:73-79. DOI: http://dx.doi.org/10.1016/S0020-7519(00)00148-X

[33] Kahn C, Line S. The Merck Veterinary Manual. Merck and Company Inc. New Jersey, USA. Giardiasis; 2010; pp. 190-192; 170. ISBN-13: 978-0911910933; ISBN-10: 091191093X

[34] Chin HS, Palm D, McArthur AG, Svärd SG, Gillin FD. A novel Myb-related protein involved in transcriptional activation of encystation genes in *Giardia lamblia*. Clinical Microbiology. 2002;**46**:971-984. DOI: 10.1046/j.1365-2958.2002.03233.x

[35] Eckmann L. Mucosal defenses against *Giardia*. Parasite Immunology. 2003;**25**:259-270. DOI: 10.1046/j.1365-3024.2003.00634.x

[36] O'Handley R, Cockwill C, McAllister T, Jelinski M, Morck D, Olson M. Duration of naturally acquired giardiosis and cryptosporidiosis in dairy calves and their association with diarrhoea. Journal of the American Veterinary Medical Association. 1999;**214**:391-396 10023403

[37] Ralston B, McAllister T, Olson M. Prevalence and infection pattern of naturally acquired giardiasis and cryptosporidiosis in range beef calves and their dams. Veterinary Parasitology. 2003;**114**:113-122. DOI: http://dx.doi.org/10.1016/S0304-4017(03)00134-1

[38] Xiao L, Herd RP. Epidemiology of equine *Cryptosporidium* and *Giardia* infections. Equine Veterinary Journal. 1994;**26**:14-17. DOI: 10.1111/j.2042-3306.1994.tb04323.x

[39] Becher K, Robertson I, Fraser D, Palmer D, Thompson R. Molecular epidemiology of *Giardia* and *Cryptosporidium* infections in dairy calves originating from three sources in Western Australia. Veterinary Parasitology. 2004;**123**:19. DOI: http://dx.doi.org/10.1016/j.vetpar.2004.05.020

[40] Appelbee A, Thompson R, Olson E. *Giardia* and *Cryptosporidium* in mammalian wildlife-current status and future needs. Trends in Parasitology. 2005;**21**:370-376. DOI: http://dx.doi.org/10.1016/j.pt.2005.06.004

[41] Thompson RC, Carlysle S, Palmer CS, O'Handley, R. The public health and clinical significance of *Giardia* and *Cryptosporidium* in domestic animals. The Veterinary Journal. 2008;**177**:18-25. DOI: http://dx.doi.org/10.1016/j.tvjl.2007.09.022

[42] Geurden T, Claerebout E, Dursin L, Deflandre A, Bernay F, Kaltsatos V, Vercruysse J. The efficacy of an oral treatment with paromomycin against an experimental infection with *Giardia* in calves. Veterinary Parasitology. 2006;**135**:241247. DOI: http://dx.doi.org/10.1016/j.vetpar.2005.09.006

[43] Olson M, McAllister T, Deselliers L, Morck D, Cheng K, Buret A, Ceri H. Effects of giardiasis on production in a domestic ruminant (lamb) model. American Journal of Veterinary Research. 1995;**56**:1470-1474 8585658

[44] Huetink R, van der Giessen J, Noordhuizen J, Ploeger H. Epidemiology of *Cryptosporidium* spp. and *Giardia duodenalis* on a dairy farm. Veterinary Parasitology. 2001;**102**:53-67. DOI: http://dx.doi.org/10.1016/S0304-4017(01)00514-3

[45] Xiao L. *Giardia* infection in farm animals. Parasitology Today 1994;**10**:436-438. DOI: https://doi.org/10.1016/0169-4758(94)90178-3

[46] O'Handley RM. *Giardia* in farm animals. In: Olson BE, Olson ME, Wallis PM, editors. *Giardia*: The Cosmopolitan Parasite. Wallingford, UK: CAB International; 2002. p. 97-105

[47] Sabry M, Taher E, Meabed E. Prevalence and genotyping of zoonotic *Giardia* from Fayoum Governorate, Egypt. Research Journal of Parasitology. 2009;**4**:105-114. ISSN: 1816-4943

[48] Di Cristanziano V, Santoro M, Parasi F, Albonico M, Shaali M, Di Cave D, Berrilli F. Genetic characterization of *Giardia duodenalis* by sequence analysis in humans and animals in Pemba Island, Tanzania. Parasitology International 2013;**63**:438-441. DOI: http://dx.doi.org/10.1016/j.parint.2013.11.004

[49] Helmy YA, Krücken J, Nöckler K, Samson-Himmelstjerna G, Zessin GH. Comparison between two commercially available serological tests and polymerase chain reaction in the diagnosis of *Cryptosporidium* in animals and diarrhoeic children. Parasitology Research. 2014;**113**:211. DOI: 10.1007/s00436-013-3645-3

[50] Kakandelwa C, Siwila J, Nalubamba KS, Muma JB, Phiri IGK. Prevalence of *Giardia* in dairy cattle in Lusaka and Chilanga districts, Zambia. Veterinary Parasitology. 2016;**215**:114-116. DOI: http://dx.doi.org/10.1016/j.vetpar.2015.11.004

[51] Trout J, Santı'n M, Greiner E, Fayer R. Prevalence and genotypes of *Giardia duodenalis* in post-weaned dairy calves. Veterinary Parasitology. 2005;**130**:177-183. DOI: http://dx.doi.org/10.1016/j.vetpar.2005.03.032

[52] Mendonca C, Almeida A, Castro A, de Lurdes Delgado M, Soares S, da Costa, M, et al. Molecular characterization of *Cryptosporidium* and *Giardia* isolates from cattle from Portugal. Veterinary Parasitology 2007;**147**:47-50. DOI: http://dx.doi.org/10.1016/j.vetpar.2007.03.019

[53] Monis T, Andrews H, Mayrhofer G, Ey L. Genetic diversity within the morphological species *Giardia intestinalis* and its relationship to host origin. Infection, Genetics and Evolution. 2003;**3**:29-38. DOI: http://dx.doi.org/10.1016/S1567-1348(02)00149-1.

[54] Thompson RC, Monis PT. Variation in *Giardia*: Implications for taxonomy and epidemiology. Advances in Parasitology. 2004;**58**: 69-137. DOI: http://dx.doi.org/10.1016/S0065-308X(04)58002-8

[55] Sischo WM, Atwill ER, Lanyon LE, George J. Cryptosporidia on dairy farms and the role that these farms may have in contaminating surface water supplies in the Northeastern United States. Preventive Veterinary Medicine, 2000;**43**:253-267. DOI: http://dx.doi.org/10.1016/S0167-5877(99)00107-5

[56] Ryan UM, Bath C, Robertson I, Read C, Elliot A, McInnes L, Traub R, Besier B. Sheep may not be an important zoonotic reservoir for *Cryptosporidium* and *Giardia* parasites. Applied Environmental Microbiology. 2005;**71**:4992-4997. DOI: 10.1128/AEM.71.9.4992-4997.2005

[57] Castro-Hermida JA, Almeid A, Gonzalez-Warleta M, Da Costa JM, Mezo M. Prevalence and preliminary genetic analysis of *Giardia* isolated from adult sheep in Galicia (northwest Spain). Journal of Eukaryotic Microbiology. 2006;**53**(Suppl 1):S172-S173. DOI: 10.1111/j.1550-7408.2006.00220.x

[58] Castro-Hermida JA, Almeida A, Gonzalez-Warleta M, Correia da Costa JM, Rumbo Lorenzo C, Mezo M. Occurrence of *Cryptosporidium parvum* and *Giardia duodenalis* in healthy adult domestic ruminants. Parasitology Research. 2007;**101**:1443-1448. DOI: 10.1007/s00436-007-0624-6

[59] Santı'n M, Trout JM, Fayer R. Prevalence and molecular characterization of *Cryptosporidium* and *Giardia* species and genotypes in sheep in Maryland. Veterinary Parasitology. 2007;**146**:17-24. DOI: http://dx.doi.org/10.1016/j.vetpar.2007.01.010

[60] Wegayehu T, MdR K, Li J, Adamu H, Erko B, Zhang L, Tilahun G. Prevalence and genetic characterization of *Cryptosporidium* species and *Giardia duodenalis* in lambs in Oromia Special Zone, Central Ethiopia. BMC Veterinary Research. 2017;**13**:22. DOI: 10.1186/s12917-016-0916-0

[61] Wang H, Qi M, Zhang K, Li J, Huang J, Ning C, Zhang L. Prevalence and genotyping of *Giardia duodenalis* isolated from sheep in Henan Province, central China. Infection, Genetics and Evolution. 2016;**39**:330-335. DOI: http://dx.doi.org/10.1016/j.meegid.2016.02.006

[62] Olson M, Thorlakson C, Deselliers L, Morck D, McAllister T. *Giardia* and *Cryptosporidium* in Canadian farm animals. Veterinary Parasitology, 1997;**68**,375-381. DOI: http://dx.doi.org/10.1016/S0304-4017(96)01072-2

[63] Paz e Silva FM, Lopes RS, Bresciani KDS, Amarante AFT, Araujo JP Jr. High occurrence of *Cryptosporidium ubiquitum* and *Giardia duodenalis* genotype E in sheep from Brazil. Acta Parasitologica. 2014;**59**:193-196. DOI: 10.2478/s11686-014-0223-5

[64] Ye J, Xiao L, Wang Y, Guo Y, Roellig DM, Feng Y. Dominance of *Giardia duodenalis* assemblage A and Enterocytozoon bieneusi genotype BEB6 in sheep in Inner Mongolia, China. Veterinary Parasitology 2015;**210**:235-239. DOI: http://dx.doi.org/10.1016/j.vetpar.2015.04.011

[65] Yang R, Jacobson C, Gordon C, Ryan U. Prevalence and molecular characterization of *Cryptosporidium* and *Giardia* species in pre-weaned sheep in Australia. Veterinary Parasitology 2009;**161**:19-24. DOI: http://dx.doi.org/10.1016/j.vetpar.2008.12.021

[66] Giangaspero A, Paoletti B, Iorio R, Traversa D. Prevalence and molecular characterization of *Giardia duodenalis* from sheep in central Italy. Parasitology Research. 2005;**96**:32-37. DOI: 10.1007/s00436-005-1317-7

[67] Geurden T, Thomas P, Casaert S, Vercruysse J, Claerebout E. Prevalence and molecular characterization of *Cryptosporidium* and *Giardia* in lambs and goat kids in Belgium. Veterinary Parasitology. 2008;**155**:142-145. DOI: http://dx.doi.org/10.1016/j.vetpar.2008.05.002

[68] Van der Giessen JW, de Vries A, Roos M, Wielinga P, Kortbeek LM, Mank TG. Genotyping of *Giardia* in Dutch patients and animals: A phylogenetic analysis of human and animal isolates. International Journal of Parasitology 2006;**36**:849-858. DOI: 10.1016/j.ijpara.2006.03.001

[69] Aloisio F, Filippini G, Antenucci P, Lepri E, Pezzotti G, Caccio SM, Pozio E. Severe weight loss in lambs infected with *Giardia duodenalis* assemblage B. Veterinary Parasitology. 2006;**142**:154-158. DOI: 10.1016/j.vetpar.2006.06.023

[70] Appelbee AJ, Frederick LM, Heitman TL, Olson ME. Prevalence and genotyping of *Giardia duodenalis* from beef calves in Alberta, Canada. 2003;**112**:289-294. DOI: http://dx.doi.org/10.1016/S0304-4017(02)00422-3

[71] Ruiz A, Foronda P, Gonzalez JF, Guedes A, Abreu-Acosta N, Molina JM, Valladares B. Occurrence and genotype characterization of *Giardia duodenalis* in goat kids from the Canary Islands, Spain. Veterinary Parasitology. 2008;**154**:137-141. DOI: http://dx.doi.org/10.1016/j.vetpar.2008.03.003

[72] Berilli F, D'Alfonso R, Giangaspero A, Marangi M, Brandonisio O, Kabore Y, Gle C, Cianfanelli C, Lauro R, Cave D. *Giardia duodenalis* genotypes and *Cryptosporidium* species in humans and domestic animals in Côte dÍvoire: Occurrence and evidence for environmental contamination. Transactions of the Royal Society of Tropical Medicine and Hygiene. 2012;**106**:191-195. DOI: http://dx.doi.org/10.1016/j.trstmh.2011.12.005

[73] Lim YAL, Mahdy MAK, Tan TK, Goh XT, Jex AR, Nolan MJ, Sharma RSK, Gasser RB. First molecular characterization of *Giardia duodenalis* from goats in Malaysia. Molecular and Cellular Probes 2013;**27**:28-31. DOI: http://dx.doi.org/10.1016/j.mcp.2012.08.006

[74] Akinkuotu OA, Okwelum N, Famakinde SA, Akinkuotu AC, Oseni OT. *Giardia* infection in recently acclimatized kalahari red goats in Nigeria. Nigerian Veterinary Journal. 2016;**37**:16-23 ISSN 0331-3026

[75] Robertson LJ. *Giardia* and *Cryptosporidium* infections in sheep and goats: A review of the potential for transmission to humans via environmental contamination. Epidemiology and Infection. 2009;**137**:913-921. DOI: 10.1017/S0950268809002295

[76] Gomez-Munoz MT, Navarro C, Garijo-Toledo MM, Dea-Ayuela MA, Fernandez-Barredo S, Perez-Gracia MT, Dominguez-Marquez MV, Borras R. Occurrence and genotypes of *Giardia* isolated from lambs in Spain. Parasitology International 2009;**58**:297-299. DOI: http://dx.doi.org/10.1016/j.parint.2009.06.005

[77] Zhang W, Zhang X, Wang R, Liu A, Shen Y, Ling H, Cao J, Yang F, Zhang X, Zhang L. Genetic characterizations of *Giardia duodenalis* in sheep and goats in Heilongjiang Province, China and possibility of zoonotic transmission. PLoS Neglected Tropical Disease. 2012;**6**:e1826. DOI: http://dx.doi.org/10.1371/journal.pntd.0001826

[78] Sanford SE. Enteric cryptosporidial infection in pigs: 184 cases (1981-1985). Journal of the American Veterinary Medical Association. 1987;**190**:695-698. PMID:3570923

[79] Koudela B, Nohynkova E, Vitovec J, Pakandl M, Kulda J. *Giardia* infections in pigs: Detection and in vitro isolation if trophozoites of the *Giardia intestinalis* group. Parasitology 1991;**102**:163-166. DOI: http://dx.doi.org/10.1017/S0031182000062442

[80] Xiao L, Herd RP, Bowman GL. Prevalence of *Cryptosporidium* and *Giardia* infections on two Ohio pig farms with different management systems. Veterinary Parasitology. 1994;**52**: 331-336. DOI: http://dx.doi.org/10.1016/0304-4017(94)90124-4

[81] Atwill ER, Sweitzer RA, Pereira MG, Gardner IA, Van Vuren D, Boyce WM. Prevalence of and associated risk factors for shedding *Cryptosporidium parvum* oocysts and *Giardia* cysts within feral pig populations in California. Applied and Environmental Microbiology. 1997;**63**:3946-3949 0099-2240/97/$04.0010. ISSN: 1098-5336

[82] Farzan A, Parrington L, Coklin T, Cook A, Pintar K, Pollari F, Friendship R, Farber J, Dixon B. Detection and characterization of *Giardia duodenalis* and *Cryptosporidium* spp. on swine farms in Ontario, Canada. Foodborne Pathogens and Disease. 2011;**8**:1207-1213

[83] Maddox-Hyttel C, Langkjaer RB, Enemark HL, Vigre H. *Cryptosporidium* and *Giardia* in different age groups of Danish cattle and pigs – Occurrence and management of associated risk factors. Veterinary Parasitology. 2006;**141**:48-59 http://dx.doi.org/10.1016/j.vetpar.2006.04.032, PMID: 16797848

[84] Hamnes I, Gjerde B, Forberg T, Robertson L. Occurrence of *Cryptosporidium* and *Giardia* in suckling piglets in Norway. Veterinary Parasitology. 2007;**144**:222-233. DOI: http://dx.doi.org/10.1016/j.vetpar.2006.10.011

[85] Langkjaer RB, Vigre H, Enemark HL, Maddox-Hyttel C. Molecular and phylogenetic characterization of *Cryptosporidium* and *Giardia* from pigs and cattle in Denmark. Parasitology. 2007;**134**:339-350. DOI: 10.1017/S0031182006001533

[86] Siwila J, Mwape KE. Prevalence of *Cryptosporidium* spp. and *Giardia duodenalis* in pigs in Lusaka, Zambia. Onderstepoort Journal of Veterinary Research. 2012;**79**:5 pages, Art. #404. DOI: http://dx.doi.org/10.4102/ojvr.v79i1.404

[87] Armson A, Yang R, Thompson J, Johnson J, Reid S, Ryan UM. *Giardia* genotypes in pigs in Western Australia: prevalence and association with diarrhoea. Experimental Parasitology. 2009;**121**:381-383. DOI: 10.1016/j.exppara.2009.01.008

[88] Sprong H, Caccio SM, van der Giessen JW. Identification of zoonotic genotypes of *Giardia duodenalis*. PLoS Neglected Tropical Diseases. 2009;**3**:e558. DOI: http://dx.doi.org/10.1371/journal.pntd.0000558

[89] Xiao L, Fayer R. Molecular characterisation of species and genotypes of *Cryptosporidium* and *Giardia* and assessment of zoonotic transmission. International Journal of Parasitology 2008;38:1239-1255. DOI: http://dx.doi.org/10.1016/j.ijpara.2008.03.006

[90] Traub RJ. The veterinary public health significance of *Giardia* and *Cryptosporidium*: getting things in perspective. Veterinary Journal. 2008;**177**:309-310. DOI: 10.1016/j.tvjl.2008.06.013

[91] Claerebout E, Casaert S, Dalemans AC, De Wilde N, Levecke B, Vercruysse J, Geurden T. *Giardia* and other intestinal parasites in different dog populations in Northern Belgium. Veterinary Parasitology. 2009;161:41-46. DOI: http://dx.doi.org/10.1016/j.vetpar.2008.11.024

[92] Bouzid M, Halai K, Jeffreys D, Hunter PR. The prevalence of *Giardia* infection in dogs and cats: a systematic review and meta-analysis of prevalence studies from stool samples. Veterinary Parasitology. 2015;**207**:181-202. DOI: 10.1016/j.vetpar.2014.12.011

[93] Stehr-Green JK, Murray G, Schantz PM, Wahlquist SP. Intestinal parasites in pet store puppies in Atlanta. American Journal of Public Health. 1987;**77**:345-346. DOI: 10.2105/AJPH.77.3.345

[94] Papini G, Gorini A, Spaziani R, Cardini G. Survey on giardiasis in shelter dog populations. Veterinary Parasitology. 2005;**128**:333-339. DOI: http://dx.doi.org/10.1016/j.vetpar.2004.12.005

[95] Dubná S, Langrova J, Napravnik I, Jankovska J, Vadlejch Pekar S, Fechtner J. The prevalence of intestinal parasites in dogs from Prague, rural areas, and shelters of the Czech Republic. Veterinary Parasitology. 2007;**145**:120-128. DOI: http://dx.doi.org/10.1016/j.vetpar.2006.11.006

[96] Mark-Carew MP, Adesiyun AA, Basu A, Georges KA, Pierre T, Tilitz S, Wade SE, Mohammed HO. Characterization of *Giardia duodenalis* infections in dogs in Trinidad and Tobago. Veterinary Parasitology. 2013;**196**:199-202. DOI: http://dx.doi.org/10.1016/j.vetpar.2013.01.023

[97] Bugg RJ, Robertson ID, Elliot AD, Thompson RCA. Gastrointestinal parasites of urban dogs in Perth, Western Australia. Veterinary Journal. 1999;**157**:295-301. DOI: https://doi.org/10.1053/tvjl.1998.0327

[98] McGlade TR, Robertson ID, Elliott AD, Thompson RCA. High prevalence of *Giardia* detected in cats by PCR. Veterinary Parasitology. 2003;**110**:197-205. DOI: http://dx.doi.org/10.1016/S0304-4017(02)00322-9

[99] Thompson RCA, Robertson ID. Gastrointestinal parasites of dogs and cats: current issues. Compendium on continuing education for the practising. The Veterinarian. 2003;**25**:4-11

[100] Ballweber LR, Xiao L, Bowman DD, Kahn G, Cama VA. Giardiasis in dogs and cats: update on epidemiology and public health significance. Trends in Parasitology. 2010;**26**:180-189. DOI: http://dx.doi.org/10.1016/j.pt.2010.02.005

[101] Traub RJ, Monis P, Robertson I, Irwin P, Mencke N, Thompson RCA. Epidemiological and molecular evidence supports the zoonotic transmission of *Giardia* among humans and dogs living in the same community. Parasitology. 2004;**128**:253-262. DOI: 10.1017/S0031182003004505

[102] Volotao AC, Costa-Macedo L M, Haddad FS, Brandao A, Peralta JM, Fernandes O. Genotyping of *Giardia duodenalis* from human and animal samples from Brazil using beta-giardin gene: A phylogenetic analysis. Acta Tropica 2007;**102**:10-19. DOI: http://dx.doi.org/10.1016/j.actatropica.2007.02.010

[103] Traub R, Inpankaew T, Reid S, Sutthikornchai C, Sukthana Y, Robertson I, Thompson R. Transmission cycles of *Giardia duodenalis* in dogs and humans in Temple communities

of Bangkok – A critical evaluation of its prevalence using three diagnostic tests in the field in the absence of a gold standard. Acta Tropica. 2009;**111**:125132. DOI: http://dx.doi.org/10.1016/j.actatropica.2007.02.010

[104] Covacin C, Aucoin DP, Elliot A, Thompson RC. Genotypic characterisation of *Giardia* from domestic dogs in the USA. VeterinaryParasitology. 2011;**177**:2832. DOI: http://dx.doi.org/10.1016/j.vetpar.2010.11.029

[105] Farthing MJG. Giardiasis as a disease. In: Thompson RCA, Reynoldson JA, Lymbery AJ, editors. *Giardia*: From Molecules to Disease. Wallingford, England: CAB International; 1994. pp. 15-37

[106] Robertson ID, Irwin PJ, Lymbery AJ, Thompson RCA. The role of companion animals in the emergence of parasitic zoonoses', International Journal of Parasitology. 2000;**30**:13691377. DOI: http://dx.doi.org/10.1016/S0020 7519(00)00134-X

[107] Fantham HB. Some parasitic protozoa found in South Africa: IV. South African Journal of Science. 1921;**18**:164170. ISSN: 0038-2353

[108] Bemrick W. *Giardia* in North American horses. Veterinary Medicine Small Animal Clinics. 1968;**63**:163-165. PMID:5185280

[109] Atwill ER, McDougald NK, Perea L. Cross-sectional study of faecal shedding of *Giardia duodenalis* and *Cryptosporidium parvum* among packstock in the Sierra Nevada Range. Equine Veterinary Journal. 2000;**32**:247-252. DOI: 10.2746/042516400776563545

[110] Veronesi F, Passamonti F, Caccio S, Diaferia M, Fioretti DP. Epidemiological survey on equine *Cryptosporidium* and *Giardia* infections in Italy and molecular characterization of isolates. Zoonoses and Public Health. 2010;**57**:510-517. DOI: 10.1111/j.1863-2378.2009.01261.x

[111] Manahan FF. Diarrhoea in horses with particular reference to a chronic diarrhoea syndrome. Australian Veterinary Journal. 1970;**46**:231-234. DOI: 10.1111/j.1751-0813.1970.tb02014.x

[112] Kirkpatrick CE, Skand DL. Giardiasis in a horse. Journal of the American Veterinary Medical Association. 1985;**187**:163-164. PMID:4030452

[113] Pavlásek I, Hess L, Stehlik I, Stika V. The first detection of *Giardia* spp. in horses in the Czech Republic. Veterinární Medicína. 1995;**40**:81-86. PMID:7762123

[114] Beelitz P, Göbel E, Gothe R. Spectrum of species and incidence of endoparasites in foals and their mother mares from breeding farms with and without anthelmintic prophylaxis in upper Bavaria. Tierarztliche Praxis. 1996;**24**:48-54. PMID: 8720956 (Abstract)

[115] Johnson E, Atwill ER, Filkins ME, Kalush J. The prevalence of shedding of *Cryptosporidium* and *Giardia* spp. based on a single fecal sample collection from each of 91 horses used for backcountry recreation. Journal of Veterinary Diagnostic Investigation. 1997;**9**:56-60

[116] Traub R, Wade S, Read C, Thompson A, Mohammed H. Molecular characterization of potentially zoonotic isolates of *Giardia duodenalis* in horses. Veterinary Parasitology 2005;**130**:317-321. DOI: http://dx.doi.org/10.1016/j.vetpar.2005.02.011

[117] Traversa D, Otranto D, Milillo P, Latrofa MS, Giangaspero A, Di Cesare A, Paoletti B. *Giardia duodenalis* sub-Assemblage of animal and human origin in horses. Infection, Genetics and Evolution 2012;**12**:1642-1646. DOI: http://dx.doi.org/10.1016/j.meegid.2012.06.014

[118] Monis PT, Andrews RH, Mayrhofer G, Ey PL. Molecular systematics of the parasitic protozoan *Giardia intestinalis*. Molecular Biology and Evolution. 1999;**16**:1135-1144. DOI: https://doi.org/10.1093/oxfordjournals.molbev.a026204

[119] Zajac AM, Johnson J, King SE. Evaluation of the importance of centrifugation as a component of zinc sulfate fecal flotation examinations. Journal of American Animal Hospital Association. 2002;**38**:221-224. DOI: http://dx.doi.org/10.5326/0380221

[120] Garcia LS. Diagnostic Medical Parasitology. 5th ed. Washington, DC: ASM press; 2007. pp. 813-816

[121] Addis DG, Mathews HM, Stewart JM, Walquist SP, Williams RM, Finton RJ, Spencer HC, Juranek DD. Evaluation of a commercially available enzyme linked immunosorbent assay for *Giardia lamblia* antigen in stool. Journal of Clinical Microbiology. 1991;**29**:1137-1142 0095-1137/91/061137-06$02.00/0. PMCID: PMC269958

[122] Farthing MJG. Giardiasis. In: Gills HM, editor. Edns Protozoal Diseases. UK: Arnold Publishers; 1999. p. 562-584

[123] Tangtrongsup S. Update on the diagnosis and management of *Giardia* spp infections in dogs and cats. Topics in Companion Animal Medicine. 2010;**25**:155-162. DOI: 10.1053/j.tcam.2010.07.003

[124] Caccio S, De Giacomo M, Pozio E. Sequence analysis of the b-giardin gene and development of a polymerase chain reaction-restriction fragment length polymorphism assay to genotype *Giardia duodenalis* cysts from human faecal samples. International Journal for Parasitology 2002;**32**:1023-1030. DOI: http://dx.doi.org/10.1016/S0020-7519(02)00068-1

[125] Chalmers RM. Advances in diagnosis: Is microscopy still the benchmark? In: Ortega-Pierres G, Caccio S, Fayer R, Mank TG, Smith HV, Thompson RCA, editors. *Giardia* and *Cryptosporidium*, from molecules to disease. CAB International. 2009; pp. 147-157. ISBN: 13:978 1 84593 391 3

[126] Savioli L, Smith H, Thompson A. *Giardia* and *Cryptosporidium* join the 'Neglected Diseases Initiative'. Trends in Parasitology. 2006;**22**:203-208. DOI: http://dx.doi.org/10.1016/j.pt.2006.02.015

[127] Xiao L, Saeed K, Herd RP. Efficacy of albendazole and fenbendazole against *Giardia* infec tion in cattle. Veterinary Parasitology. 1996;**61**:165. DOI: https://doi.org/10.1016/0304-4017(95)00802-0

[128] Garossino KC, Ralston BJ, McAllister TA, Milligan DN, Royan G, Olson ME. Individual intake and antiparasitic efficacy of free choice mineral and fenbendazole in range calves. Veterinary Parasitology. 2001;**94**:151. DOI: http://dx.doi.org/10.1016/S0304-4017(00)00380-0

[129] O'Handley R M, Cockwill C, Jelinski M, McAllister TA, Olson ME. Effects of repeat fenbendazole treatment in dairy calves with giardiosis on cyst excretion, clinical signs and production. Veterinary Parasitology. 2000;**89**:209-218. DOI: http://dx.doi.org/10.1016/S0304-4017(00)00200-4

[130] Stokol T, Randolph JF, Nachbar S, Rodi C, Barr SC. Development of bone marrow toxicosis after albendazole administration in a dog and cat. Journal American Veterinary Medical Association. 1997;**210**:1753-1756 9187723

[131] Olson ME, Ceri H, Morck DW. *Giardia* vaccination. Parasitology Today. 2000;**16**:213-217. DOI: http://dx.doi.org/10.1016/S0169-4758(99)01623-3

[132] Montoya A, Dado D, Mateo M, Espinosa C, Miró G. Efficacy of Drontal®flavour Plus (50 mg praziquantel 144 mg pyrantel embonate, 150 mg febantelper tablet) against *Giardia* sp. in naturally infected dogs. Parasitology Research. 2008;**103**:1141-1144. DOI: 10.1007/s00436-008-1107-0

Section 2

Biological and Diagnostic Aspects

Chapter 5

The Cytoskeleton of *Giardia intestinalis*

Ana Paula Rocha Gadelha, Marlene Benchimol and Wanderley de Souza

Additional information is available at the end of the chapter

http://dx.doi.org/10.5772/intechopen.70243

Abstract

Giardia intestinalis is a pathogenic protozoan, which is the causative agent of giardiasis. The *Giardia* trophozoite presents a cytoskeleton formed by specialized microtubular structures such as the ventral disk, four pairs of flagella, the median body, and the *funis* that are involved in cell division and differentiation. Because trophozoite motility and adhesion to the host intestinal cells are important processes mediated by the parasite cytoskeleton, the fine regulation of these elements may be directly related to the mechanisms that underlie infection. The organization of *Giardia* cytoskeleton at the ultrastructural level has been analyzed by different classical microscopy methods, including negative stain and chemical fixation for scanning and transmission electron microscopy. In this chapter, we provide an overview of the *G. intestinalis* cytoskeleton, emphasizing its structural organization and proteins involved in the maintenance of the structures as well as their functional role. These structures have been recently analyzed in some detail using techniques such as electron microscopy tomography, cryoelectron microscopy, ultra-high resolution scanning electron microscopy (UHRSEM), and helium ion microscopy (HIM). In addition, genome survey and phylogenetic analysis as well as proteomic analysis have revealed the presence of several new and not yet well-characterized proteins.

Keywords: *Giardia intestinalis*, cytoskeleton, ventral disk, flagella, median body, *funis*, microfilaments

1. Introduction

Giardia intestinalis (also known as *Giardia lamblia* and *Giardia duodenalis*) is a flagellated protist described for the first time in 1681 by Antony Van Leeuwenhoek, after a discovery he made while examining his own feces using a primitive light microscope. This species is the causative agent of a parasitic disease known as giardiasis, an intestinal illness characterized by chronic diarrhea and undernutrition [1]. Giardiasis is a waterborne disease with a worldwide distribution [2].

Approximately, 200 million people are currently infected with *G. intestinalis.* The prevalence of giardiasis is higher in areas where sanitation conditions are inadequate. The illness mainly affects children and immunocompromised individuals. The life cycle of *G. intestinalis* comprises of two developmental stages: the trophozoite, in which it inhabits the host's small intestine, and the cyst, in which it is immobile and resistant to stress conditions of the environmental milieu [3]. A more detailed description of basic biological aspects of this protozoan is presented in another chapter of this book. Host infection begins after ingestion of cysts present in contaminated water or food. When a cyst is subjected to the acidic pH and gastric enzymes of the stomach, a reorganization of the cyst wall takes place initiating the encystment process. Each cyst will differentiate into two trophozoites [4]. This process ends in the duodenum through the proteolytic action of pancreatic enzymes (specifically, chymotrypsin and trypsin) and alkalinization on the cyst wall [5]. When released into the small intestine, the trophozoites penetrate the intestinal mucus layer and attach to the epithelium of the duodenum and the upper jejunum. After division by binary fission, they form a monolayer that covers the entire intestinal surface. Some researchers have suggested that the physical attachment of *Giardia* trophozoites to the host intestinal epithelium may contribute to structural and functional changes in the host intestinal cells [6, 7]. Analysis of the *Giardia*-host cell interactions *in vitro* shows that this parasite is responsible for an increase in intestinal permeability due to the rearrangement of proteins of the tight adherens and desmosomal junctions [8–10]. Here, we will focus on the cytoskeleton of the trophozoite, which presents a half-pear shape with a bilateral symmetry and exhibits several unusual cytoskeleton structures such as the ventral disk, the median body, the *funis*, and the lateral crest, in addition to four pairs of flagella (**Figure 1a–c**).

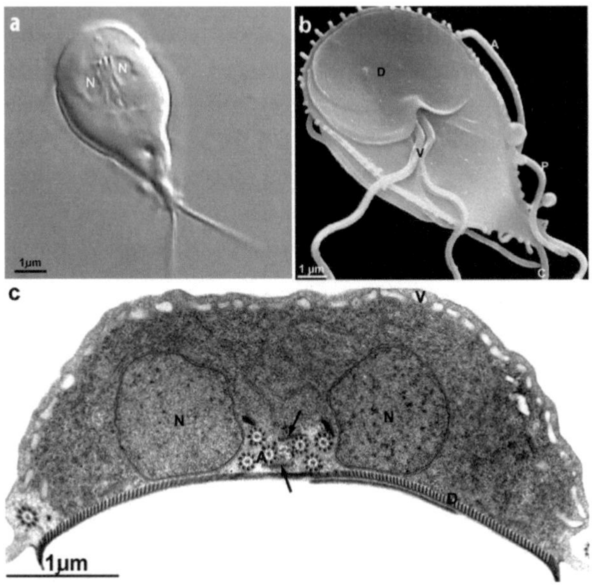

Figure 1. A general view of *G. intestinalis* trophozoites by light and electron microscopy. (a) Dorsal side of the trophozoite as observed by differential interference contrast (DIC). The two nuclei (N) are observed in the anterior region of the cell. (b) Scanning electron microscopy of the ventral side of the trophozoites. Note that the parasite displays the pairs of flagella (anterior flagella—A, posterior flagella—P, ventral flagella—V, caudal flagella—C), the ventral disk (D), and the ventro-lateral flange. (c) Routine preparation for transmission electron microscopy (TEM) of the trophozoite showing the ventral disk (D), the two nuclei (N), peripheral vesicles (V), flagellar axonemes (A) and funis (arrows) [78]. Bars = 1 μm.

The maintenance and establishment of cell shape are fundamental roles of the cytoskeleton. Since the classic work by Elmendorf et al. [11], the cytoskeleton of *Giardia* has been considered to play an essential role in the development and maintenance of the infection, mainly because its main component, the ventral disk, is indispensable for the attachment of the protozoan to the intestinal epithelial cells.

2. Cytoskeleton structures

2.1. Ventral disk

2.1.1. Structural organization

The attachment of *Giardia* trophozoites to the host intestinal epithelium is associated with a structure called ventral disk (**Figure 2a**), which is located on the ventral side and occupies two-third of the anterior region of the cell [12]. This structure is formed by a clockwise spiral layer of microtubules (**Figure 2a**) and is adjacent to the plasma membrane lining the ventral portion of the protozoan to which the microtubules are connected by small and thin filaments [13]. Observations by electron tomography show that the disk is composed of approximately 95 microtubules [14]. Trilaminar structures, known as microribbons, extend dorsally from the microtubule wall toward the cytoplasm [15] (**Figure 2b, c**). They are connected to each other by crossbridges that present a periodicity of 15–16 nm [13, 16]. Disk microtubules originate from dense bands in a region near the caudal and posterior-lateral basal bodies [16–18]. Capped microtubule ends found in this region show that these comprise minus-end areas, whereas other microtubules ending at the margin of the ventral disk are blunt and open (plus-end), suggesting a microtubule polarity [16]. Using cryo-electron tomography, Schwartz et al. [16] demonstrated that the spiral array of the ventral disk consists of microtubules ending within the ventral disk and new microtubules inserted at the inner edge near the bare area.

Observation made by several microscopy techniques shows clearly that the disk is not a homogeneous structure displaying several regions [14, 18]. High-resolution micrographs obtained by ultra-high resolution scanning electron microscope (SEM), helium ion microscopy (HIM), and cryo-electron microscopy tomography show the existence of different domains of the ventral disk [14, 18]. In a recent work, Brown et al. [14] suggested the presence of six regions. We will briefly describe each one, comparing results obtained by several groups, then add additional two regions.

The first region, designated as the dense band microtubule nucleation zone (**Figure 2a**), comprises an area of microtubules nucleation where the microtubules which continue into the disk body are assembled and another area containing a bundle of approximately 20 short microtubules [14], known as supernumerary microtubules [13], which curve slightly opposite to the main disk spiral [18] (**Figure 2a**). It is important to point out that microribbons have not been associated with the microtubules found in the dense zone [14].

The second region is the central one, also known as the "bare area" where microtubules-microribbons complexes have not been seen [19] (**Figures 2a** and **3a**). In this zone, the protrusion of the ventral disk, a projection of the ventral plasma membrane, is clearly observed [20]. When trophozoite cell membrane is extracted with detergents, the banded collars and the

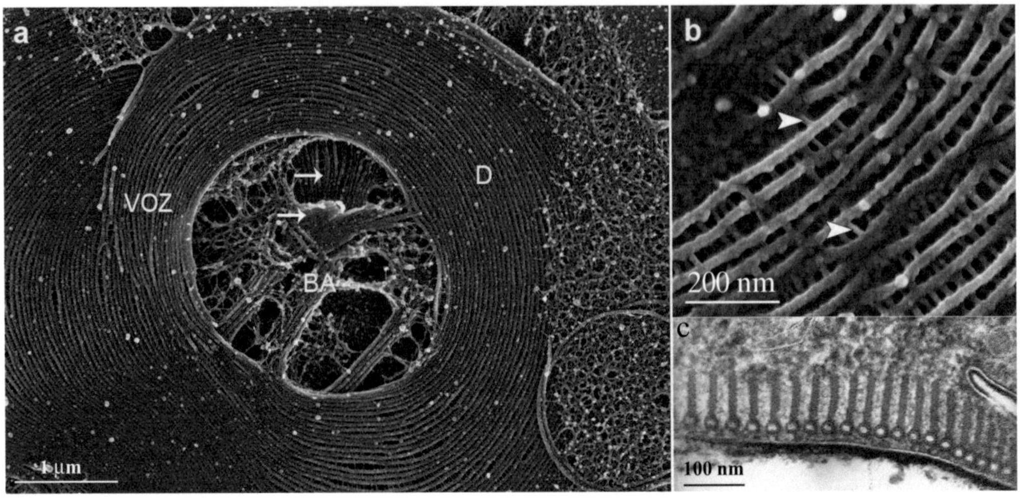

Figure 2. Cytoskeleton of *Giardia intestinalis* as observed in UHRSEM. (a) The spiral of ventral disk (D) and bare area (*) can be observed. Notice the microtubule nucleation zone with two sets of microtubules (arrows) that form the body ventral disk (D) and the ventral overlap zone (VOZ). (b, c) High magnification showing the microribbons that connect the disk microtubules (arrowheads) as seen by UHRSEM (b) and electron transmission microscopy (c) [15,18]. Bars = 1 μm.

basal bodies are observed in this region [18, 21] (**Figures 2a** and **3a**). Using ultra-high resolution scanning electron microscopy (UHRSEM) and HIM, Gadelha et al. [18] showed that there were two types of banded collars. Previously named as BC1 and BC2 [21] (**Figure 3a**), the collars were repeated on both sides of the cell. BC1 appeared as a belt-shaped structure with a thickness of 275 nm. It was associated with the basal bodies of the right caudal/posterior-lateral flagella, when cells were observed dorsally, yet associated with the left caudal/ventral flagella when the cells were observed ventrally [18] (**Figure 3b**). The BC2 was seen as a rope-shaped structure, presenting horizontal segments connected by short bridges. BC2 was continuous with the basal bodies of the left caudal/posterior-lateral flagella (dorsal view) and the right caudal/ventral flagella (ventral view) [18] (**Figure 3c**). Using electron tomography, Brown et al. [14] described this region (BC2) as a dense band composed of three distinct bands. As pointed out by Gadelha et al. [18], each BC2 presented a set of microtubules: the disk microtubules originated from the basal bodies associated with the left BC2, and the previously described supernumerary microtubules originated from the basal bodies associated with the right BC2 (**Figures 2a** and **3a**). It is not yet clear if the banded collars alone or in combination with the basal bodies could work as microtubule organizing centers that would drive the formation of a new ventral disk. Feely et al. [22] observed that isolated banded collars would have the capacity to nucleate new microtubules. Using electron tomography, Brown et al. [14] demonstrated that microtubules emerged from dense bands of two or three layers of densely packed microtubules end.

The third and fourth disk regions are the dorsal and ventral overlap zones (**Figures 2a** and **3a**). Short microribbons (30–40 nm) are connected to the microtubules found in the dorsal overlap zones and the space between each microtubule is reduced (about 25 nm) [14]. In the ventral overlap zone, the microribbons are longer (50–60 nm) and the distance between the

http://dx.doi.org/10.5772/intechopen.70243

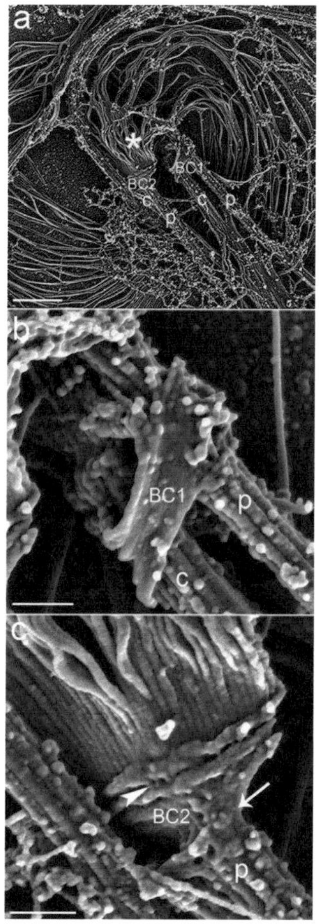

Figure 3. Dorsal view of the "bare area" of the ventral disk. (a) Axonemes of the posterior (p) and caudal (c) flagella and two banded collars (BC1 and BC2) are observed in this region. The disk microtubule (*) emerged from banded collar 2. (b) Banded collar 1 (BC1) displays a flat sheet appearance. (c) Banded collar 2 (BC2) shows horizontal segments connected by small bridges (arrowhead). These segments are continuous with the axonemes (arrow) of the left lateral-posterior (p) and caudal flagella [18]. Bars = 1 μm (a); 200 nm (b, c).

microtubules is larger (60 nm) [14]. A greater amount of microtubule-associated proteins' density, previously known as side-arms and paddles [16], is observed in the ventral zone than in the dorsal zone.

The fifth region is the disk body considered as the region where no microtubules overlap (**Figures 2a** and **3a**). At this region, the inter microtubular space is of about 70 nm, microribbons have a length of 100 nm, and the cross-bridges connecting the microtubules-microribbons complexes present a periodicity of 16 nm [14].

The sixth region is the ventral groove, which is an area located underneath the "bare area". In this region, the disk bridges are shorter and more resistant to breakage after detergent treatment, suggesting that they could be more rigid structures than those of the disk body (authors' unpublished data). As observed previously by transmission electron microscopy

[13], in the central region of the disk, overlying the slightly flattened roof of the ventral chamber, the lateral separation of the microtubules transform abruptly displaying a shorter interval between them. It is possible that the microtubules of this region are kept more closely packed due to the friction of the ventral flagella that emerges near this region and whose beating contributed to cell adhesion and motility [11, 13, 15]. The seventh region is the margin where the microtubules that nucleate at the dense band microtubule nucleation zone end. Microribbons of the marginal region of the disk are shortened and bent toward the disk center as they approach the plus-end and the margin [14]. The cross-bridges, which connect microribbons laterally, form a 16 nm axial repeats in the same way as those observed in the disk body. Volume averaging of microtubule–microribbon complexes reveals that microtubule-associated protein density and distribution in the margin are similar to the dorsal overlap zone, but much lower than in the disk body or the ventral overlap zone [14].

The eighth region is the lateral crest (**Figure 4a**), which has been described as a dense fibrous material in the periphery of ventral disk [11, 23]. As pointed by Gadelha et al. [18], this region was interconnected with the ventral disk and presented small filaments (**Figure 4b**). The low levels of cholesterol and intramembrane proteins found in this region may be associated with a great flexibility of this structure, facilitating the contraction of the outer part of the ventral disk [24]. Previous papers reported labeling for actin, myosin, α-actinin, and tropomyosin in the periphery of the ventral disk in an area that corresponded to the lateral crest [25]. Based on these observations, it was proposed that contractile activity of this region occurred during *Giardia* attachment [25]. However, recent data failed to indicate the presence of contractile proteins in the lateral crest [18, 26, 27] and demonstrated the presence of ankyrin repeat and Nek kinase domain-containing proteins [26].

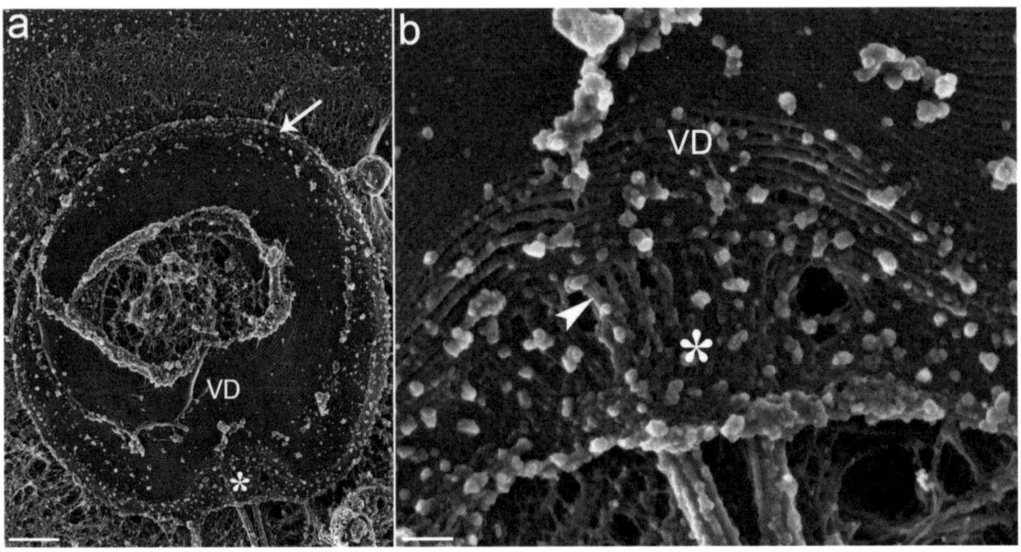

Figure 4. Lateral crest by UHRSEM. (a) The lateral crest (*) was located around the ventral disk (arrow). (b) Small filaments (arrowhead) were seen interconnecting the lateral crest (*) with the ventral disk (VD) [18]. Bars = 1 μm (a); 200 nm (b).

2.1.2. Composition

Several approaches have been used to identify the main components of the ventral disk. Since the first studies by transmission electron microscopy (TEM), it was clear that microtubules represented the major structural component of the disk. TEM studies also revealed the presence of the microribbons, another important structure. Several proteins designated as giardins have been associated with this structure. Molecular analysis demonstrated that *Giardia* has two genes for α-tubulin and three genes for β-tubulin [11, 28, 29]. *Giardia* tubulin has been described as highly modified, possibly playing a role in the stability of cytoskeleton elements. These post-translational modifications include acetylation, tyrosination, polyglycation, and polyglutamylation [30–33]. Giardin has been described as a 30 kDa protein found in microribbons and accounts for about 20% of total ventral disk protein content [34]. Several giardins have already been characterized: α-giardin, β-giardin, δ-giardin, and γ-giardin. Based on amino acid sequencing studies, α-giardins were identified as belonging to the annexin family and found in the dorsal plasma membrane of *G. intestinalis* [11, 35, 36]. One of these proteins, α-1 giardin, is a annexin with glycosaminoglycan-binding activity and is calcium-regulated [37]. However, β-giardin and δ-giardin are analogs of SF-assemblin and presumed to be present in ventral disk microribbons [11, 38, 39]. All these proteins have been shown to be associated with the various cytoskeleton structures by electrophoresis as well as by immunoblotting and immunofluorescence microscopy using specific antibodies to whole cells or to cytoskeleton preparations.

Palm et al. [40] carried out a proteomic analysis of the cytoskeleton preparation and reported the presence of a family of giardins (α-1, β, γ, and δ) and two isoforms of tubulin and a new protein, SALP-1, which is homologous to proteins that participate in the aggregation of striate fibers. Subsequently, a proteomic analysis was carried out by Lourenço et al. [41] using a cell fractionation approach. They obtained a highly enriched disk fraction that by SDS-PAGE showed the presence of five predominant bands, ranging from 25 to 58 kDa, as well as some light bands with higher molecular weight. Two-dimensional electrophoresis of the fraction revealed the presence of 18 spots. Mass spectrometry analysis of the major bands found by SDS-PAGE and of the spots identified in 2D gels revealed the presence of several additional proteins. More recently, in a seminal work Hagen et al. [26] also isolated an enriched disk fraction and used shotgun proteomics to identify its protein composition. They found 102 proteins potentially associated with the disk. In addition, several of these proteins were GFP-tagged and localized, using immunofluorescence microscopy. Six of the novel disk-associated proteins (DAPs) were localized in the whole disk in addition to those 18 previously identified [26]. Ten of the new proteins were localized in the lateral crest or along the outside edge of the ventral disk, including the Nek kinase DAP13981, a putatively contractile repetitive structure. Two novel proteins were localized in the supernumerary microtubules, which emerge from the central "bare zone" close to the flagellar basal bodies. Using the fluorescence recovery after photobleaching (FRAP) technique, evidence obtained showed that most of the identified proteins are associated with stable structures [26].

Microtubule inner proteins were also described in the ventral disk and were associated with the inner wall of the protofilaments associated with the interface microribbon-microtubules [16].

Microtubule outer proteins associated with protofilaments, localized opposite to microribbons, were also observed. A dense protein coat (previously named side-arms and paddle) of unknown composition is also observed on the margin-facing side of the microtubules [16]. In recent years, proteomic approaches combined with microscope localization technique were carried out and new disk-associated proteins were identified such as the NIMA-related kinases (Neks), ankyrin repeat domain-containing protein, median body protein, and fungal cell wall protein Mp1p. These proteins have specific sites involved in cell adhesion and TTHERM, a hypothetical protein associated with the microtubule formation in the ciliate *Tetrahymena thermophila* [26, 41]. However, despite the effort that has been made to characterize these structures by several research groups, the specific function of each of these proteins is not yet fully understood.

2.1.3. Function

The ventral disk has been considered the main structure associated with the parasite attachment to the host cell. The exact mechanism by which this occurs is still under study. In this context, several hypotheses have been raised to explain this process. Holberton's observations of the movement of the ventral flagella during cell adhesion led to the proposal of the hydrodynamic model [13, 42]. According to this theory, the suction pressure developed by the disk takes place due to the beat of the ventral flagella and the fluid flow generated by this beat through the ventro-lateral flange and the ventral groove. The authors suggested that the ventral disk would be responsible for maintaining the proper shape for creating both the suction pressure and the distance between the flange and the substrate [13, 42]. The adhesive activity of the flange was demonstrated by Hagen et al. [43]. Using interference reflection microscopy and field emission electron microscopy, these authors observed the establishment of focal contacts between the flange and the substrate [43]. Lenaghan et al. [44] showed that the ventral flagella presented a propulsive velocity of 9.4 μm/s and proposed, based on the hydrodynamic model described by [13], a suction pressure of 20.8 Pa. The main functional role of this flagella pair would then be related to the downward force required for the adhesion to the epithelium.

In contrast to the above-mentioned reports, Campanati et al. [45] suggested that the ventral flagella play a secondary role in the adhesion process. This was demonstrated with experiments where the viscosity of the medium was increased with a gradient concentration of Percoll, thereby decreasing the frequency of the flagella and checking the adhesion of the parasites. These authors found that even though the frequency of the ventral flagella decreased to about 2 Hz, many trophozoites remained adhered. They also observed contractions of the ventral disk, which consequently caused the detachment of the parasite [45]. Based on these observations, they suggested that the adhesion is not only associated with the flagellar movements; this process might also rely on other factors such as tubulin-associated movements within the ventral disk itself [45]. Using total internal reflection microscopy (TIRF) of trophozoites labeled with a fluorescent plasma membrane dye, House et al. [46] defined distinct stages of attachment: (1) skim and contact of the surface with the anterior region of the ventro-lateral flange, (2) the ventral disk periphery touches the surface, forming a continuous contact at the area of the lateral crest, (3) the lateral shield then presses the substrate, and (4) then presses the bare area region within the ventral disk. Defects in flagellar motility do not affect later stages of the attachment (steps 2–4). This was demonstrated by the generation of a strain with defects in flagellar beating by a morpholino-based knockdown of the axonemal central pair protein PF16 as well as by construction of a strain with specific defects for the ventral flagellar waveform by overexpressing a dominant negative gene. House et al. [46] observed a slower attachment during earlier stages when motility is required for positioning the ventral disk against the substrate surface (step 1). They proposed that the ventral flagellar beating might contribute to the positioning of the cell during early stages of attachment [46]. Interestingly, Woessner and Dawson [47] demonstrated that the depletion of the median body protein, a ventral disk protein, altered the domed disk conformation, and consequently, the attachment.

In addition to the mechanical mode of adhesion of this parasite to intestinal cells, as described above, other studies suggest that biochemical mechanisms involving molecular lectin-sugar interactions on the surface of *Giardia* also play an important role in this process [48]. This hypothesis was first supported by the evidence that pre-treatment of parasites with trypsin or periodate could decrease adhesion to intestinal cells. In addition, the presence of a known concentration of glucose, fucose, galactose, mannose, mannose-6-phosphate, N-acetyl-glucosamine, and N-acetyl-galactosamine in the interaction medium inhibited the attachment of the parasites to the epithelial cells [48–50]. Although these results show that lectins mediate interactions between *Giardia* and the host cell, there is a clear evidence that the cytoskeleton is sufficient to allow adhesion, as pointed out by Elmendorf et al. [11]. This conclusion is supported by the finding that trophozoites can efficiently adhere to glass, plastic, and a wide variety of mammalian cell lineages. It has been suggested that interaction of *Giardia* lectin and the carbohydrate of the intestinal cells' surface, could be important for the recognition of host duodenal cells [48].

Transmission electron microscopy analysis also showed that during cell division, the ventral disk contacts the nucleus, suggesting that this structure could cause nuclear constriction, participating in the karyokinesis process [51].

2.2. Flagella

2.2.1. Structural organization

The flagella structure of *G. intestinalis* follows the canonical 9:2+2 microtubular axoneme. The eight flagella found in the parasite are organized in pairs and are named according to their position: (1) anterior, (2) lateral-posterior, (3) ventral, and (4) caudal (**Figure 1b**). They originate from the basal bodies, which are localized between two nuclei in the anterior region of the cell [11, 17, 21].

G. intestinalis flagella present components that are associated with each pair of flagella. The axonemes of the anterior flagella extend toward the anterior region of the cell, cross to the center, and then bend running back to the posterior region where they emerge at the lateral portion of the cell. Dense fibers, named paraflagellar or paraxial rods, are associated with the intracellular portion of these axonemes [13, 18, 52] (**Figure 5a**). As observed by 3D negative staining electron tomography, striated fibers, which form a regular brush-like border, are also connected to anterior flagella [14]. The marginal plates, which have been described

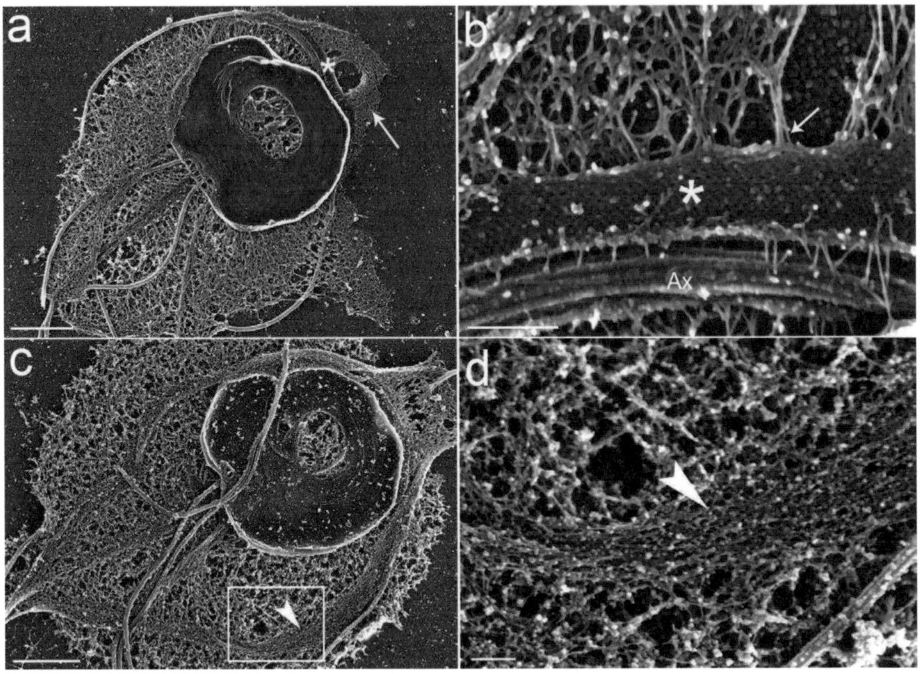

Figure 5. UHRSEM images of ventral (a–d) and dorsal surfaces of *Giardia.* (a) The marginal plates (*) are associated with a network of filaments (arrows). (b) High magnification of (a) showing the connections of the marginal plates (*) with the axoneme (Ax) and the network of filaments (arrow). (c, d) The network of filaments is continuous with the set of filaments in the periphery of the trophozoites (arrowhead). The square indicates the area in high magnification in d. (d) Note the filaments (arrowhead) parallel to the main cell axis [18]. Bars = 2 μm (a, c); 100 nm (b); 200 nm (d).

as part of the ventro-lateral flange, are also associated with the axonemes of the anterior flagella [53]. Using UHRSEM with detergent-extracted trophozoites, Maia-Brigagão et al. [52] described the fine organization of this structure. Images of the marginal plates show that they have a "boomerang-like" shape that forms an interlaced or web structure connected to the axonemes of the anterior flagella by small and apparently flexible filaments (**Figure 5b**). It has also been observed that the upper portions of the marginal plates are associated with a filamentous network in continuity with filaments that are parallel to the main cell axis [18] (**Figure 5c, d**). Together, these structures correspond to the ventro-lateral flange, which has been described as a fibrous structure of paracrystalline regularity [13, 14]. Despite the lack of biochemical information to support its functional role, the adhesive activity of the ventro-lateral flange has been suggested previously [43; see Section 2.1.3]. Dense rods are also localized just below the lateral-posterior flagella. They are shorter and associated with the inner portion of the axoneme in the region where they run along of the ventral disk [11, 54]. On the other hand, the ventral flagella are differentiated from the others by presenting a membrane projection that is filled by a dense material of unknown composition [13, 53]. A 30 kDa polypeptide was identified as the main constituent of this structure [17]. The axonemes of the caudal flagella are accompanied by two sheets of microtubules, which were called *funis* by Kulda and Nohýnková [55]. This structure will be described in more detail below.

Previous studies reported that *Giardia* flagella basal bodies were arranged in tetrads [22, 56, 57]. When the trophozoite is viewed dorsally, the left tetrad consists of anterior/ventral and caudal/posterolateral basal bodies, while the right tetrad consists of caudal/ventral and anterior/posterolateral basal bodies [56, 57]. During mitosis, association of microtubules from basal bodies with the spindle poles are thought to determine polarity of each daughter cell [58; see Section 2.6].

2.2.2. *Composition*

A number of proteins other than tubulin are found in the *G. intestinalis* flagella. Among them are the α-giardins, which have homology with human annexins and appear to have a function in trophozoite motility, adhesion, and membrane stability [59]. Interestingly, 21 α-giardin encoding genes were found in the *G. intestinalis* genome. Some members of this annexin-like protein family have been associated with the flagella. Immunocytochemical studies showed that α-2 and -19 giardin are localized in the caudal and ventral flagella, respectively [60]. An α-14 giardin that exhibits a calcium-dependent phospholipid-binding site resides at local slubs near the proximal part and the ends of the flagella, and associates with tubulin [61, 62]. Ankyrin repeats (such as GSP-180) have also been described and shown to contain coiled-coil domains and are found in the axoneme of the anterior flagellum [63]. Kinesin-2 GFP fusions (*GiKIN2a* and *GiKIN2b*) and IFT complex A and B raft homologues (IFT140 and IFT81) localize to the eight axonemes, as well as to external regions, including flagellar tips and flagellar pores [64]. Using shotgun proteomic approaches combined with GFP-tagging of microtubule-associated proteins, Hagen et al. [64] identified a homologue of DIP13, a *Chlamydomonas* protein that binds microtubules localized in the caudal and ventral flagella. γ-tubulin and centrin are located in the basal bodies of the flagella, indicating that this region could be a microtubule organizing center [65, 66] (**Figure 6**). Genomic and proteomic analysis showed that there are around 49–75 proteins localized to *Giardia* basal bodies [57, 67]. Although these proteins have been shown to be present in the flagella, it is not clear how they influence flagellar dynamics.

2.2.3. *Functions*

The *Giardia* flagella are required for motility and may be necessary for adhesion [13, 44, 45]. They participate in the emergence of the trophozoites during the excystation process [68].

Regarding the *G. intestinalis* motility, studies using video-microscopy suggest that the ventral pair beats continuously from base to the tip in a sinusoidal waveform parallel to the longitudinal axis of the cell [44, 45, 69]. The beat frequency observed in this pair of flagella was around 10 Hz, with mean amplitude of the waveform of 2.0 mm [45, 69]. Active beating is also observed in the anterior flagella, which present a beat frequency of approximately 18 Hz. Although Campanti et al. [45] have shown that the beat pattern of this pair is helical, Lenaghan et al. [44] using high-contrast and high-speed microscopic imaging (>800 fps), observed that the anterior flagella beat with a power stroke similar to ciliary motion. This same pattern was also observed during the beat of the posterior flagella [44], which was in contrast to previous analysis that suggested that the motion of the posterior flagella might be consequence of the simultaneous propagation of the waves produced by the ventral pair of the flagella [45]. The

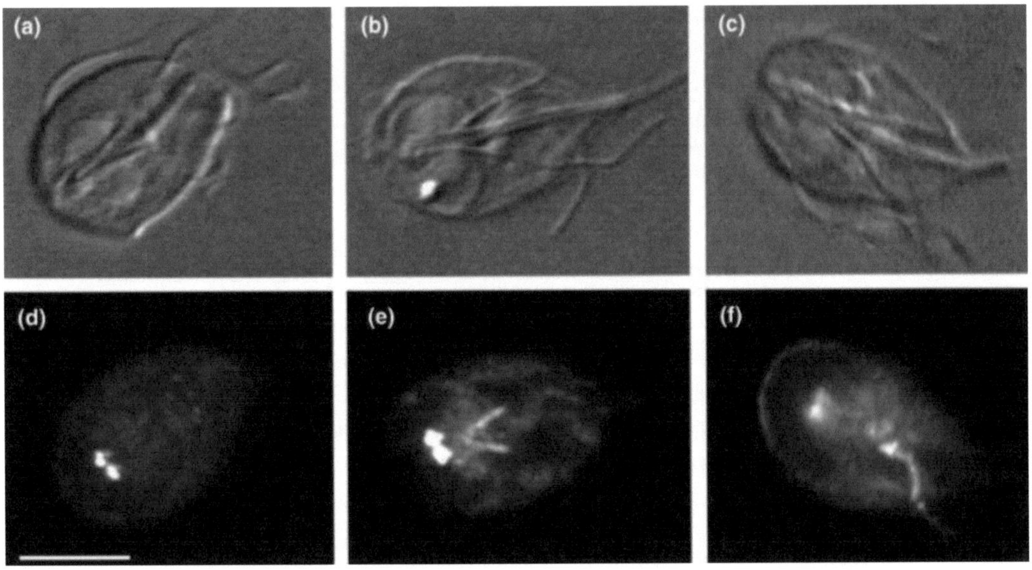

Figure 6. Presence of centrin in *G. intestinalis*. Immunostaining using anti-centrin antibodies 17E10, 2.4, and 20H5. All antibodies yielded the same labeling pattern. (a–f) Different cells are shown in differential interference contrast – DIC (a–c) and in fluorescence microscopy (d–f). Labeling is shown in the basal body, the dense rods of the posterior flagella, axonemes, flagella and disk [66]. Bars = 1 μm.

caudal pair of flagella, which emerges from the posterior end of the parasite, does not present active beating [44, 45], although motion of its intracellular portion has been observed [70].

In relation to the displacement of the trophozoite, the results found are complex. Video-microscopy observations done by Campanati et al. [45] showed that forward movement with a rocking motion was due to the beat of the anterior flagella of the cell. A change in the position of this pair of the flagella led to the rotation movement during swimming [45]. Subsequently, Lenaghan et al. [44] suggested that the fast swimming of the parasite was not the result of flagella beating, but was due to the wave-like motion of the caudal region of the cell. This movement could be the result of the active beating of the intracellular portion of the caudal flagella, which would be responsible for the dorsal-ventral flexion [44]. Another movement related to the caudal portion of the cell is lateral bending [45, 70]. This motion was observed in an early stage of attachment and was responsible for the circling swimming pattern [44]. Following the lateral flexion, a change in the direction of swimming occurs, which could be consequence of either the beating of anterior and/or ventral pair beating [44, 70].

Besides participation in the cell displacement, the *Giardia* flagella have been associated with such other cellular processes as adhesion and cell differentiation and division. Although it has been proposed that the ventral flagella beat might be essential for parasite attachment by generating a hydrodynamic force that would result in a suction-based adhesion, later studies show that this flagella pair is important in the early stages of adhesion, specifically in the positioning of the trophozoites near the substrate [45, 46; see Section 2.1.3].

The role of flagellar motility during cell differentiation and division is not yet clear. During the encystment, the flagella are not completely disarranged and flagellar movement has been observed within cysts [68]. During excystation, the flagellar motion appears to be crucial for the rupture of the cystic wall and release of the trophozoites [71]. Flagellar motility seems to be essential for the separation of daughter cells during cell division. Tumová et al. [72] showed that in the final steps of this process, the cell detaches from the substrate. During this phase, the cells are seen joined by their posterior region and swim freely in the medium while the ventral disk is assembled. Interestingly, studies using kinesin-2 mutants showed that these parasites were unable to complete cell division due to flagellar defects [73].

2.3. Median body

2.3.1. *Structural organization, composition, and function*

The median body is another microtubular element of the *G. intestinalis* cytoskeleton, but it is not present in all cells [74]. Its presence in cysts is still under discussion. It is located dorsally to the ventral disk and is between 0.2 and 1.8 μm in thickness [74]. Since its shape and position vary among species of *Giardia*, it can be used as a taxonomic tool. Previous studies have shown that the median body consists of a variable number of layers containing stable and nonstable microtubules [33, 74] (**Figure 7a–d**). Acetylated tubulin, mono and polyglycylated tubulin, and tyrosinated tubulin were detected in this structure [32, 33]. Microtubules of the median body may be associated with caudal axonemes, *funis*, plasma membrane, and occasionally, ventral disk [74] (**Figure 7a–d**). The localization of β-giardin and the presence of small bridges in these microtubules indicated that microribbons, similar to those found in the ventral disk, could be present in this structure [74, 75] (**Figure 8**). Other proteins were also described in the median body as actin and α-actinin [25]. The localization of centrin led to the suggestion that this structure could be another MTOC in *Giardia* [65, 76], although γ-tubulin has not been detected. Using green fluorescent protein-tagged microtubule-associated proteins, Dawson et al. [77] showed that kinesin-13 and EB1 localized in the median body and could play a role in the microtubular dynamic. The median body protein (MBP), a 101-kDa protein with coiled-coil domains, was initially identified in this structure. However, MBP was later identified as an abundant protein in the ventral disk, being localized in the median body of the trophozoites during prophase [47]. In this context, it was suggested that ventral disk components could assemble on the median body microtubules prior to dorsal disk biogenesis. Taken together, several hypotheses have been made for the function of the median body such as (1) microtubule reserve for rapid mobilization during mitosis and ventral disk formation; (2) microtubule organizing center; and (3) participation in the movements of the caudal region of the trophozoite [11, 74, 76].

2.4. *Funis*

2.4.1. *Structural organization, composition, and function*

The axonemes of the caudal flagella are accompanied by two sheets of microtubules, which were called *funis* by [55]. One sheet is positioned ventrally and the other dorsally [70, 78]. This microtubular complex, which contains acetylated α-tubulin [30], emanates from between the nuclei, near the region of the basal bodies, and follows until the emergence of the caudal flagella. The *funis* microtubules partially surround the axonemes of the caudal flagella and spread

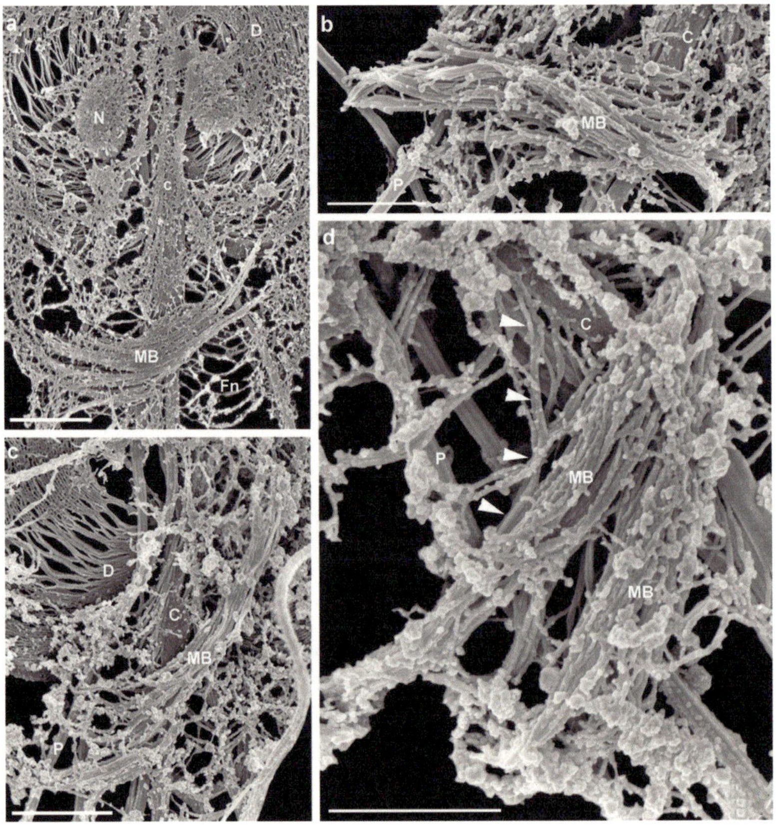

Figure 7. The FESEM of *Giardia* after detergent extraction. The plasma membrane was partially removed, allowing observation of the cytoskeleton, the MB included. The ventral disk (D), the two nuclei (N), MB, anterior (A), caudal (C) and posterior-lateral flagella (P) are seen. (a–b) Every fascicle that constitutes the MB is observed. (c–d) The median bodies are seen curved, and toward the cells' anterior region. The fascicles number is variable as well as their disposition and location. Posterior-lateral axoneme, P; caudal axoneme, C; [74]. Bars = 1 μm.

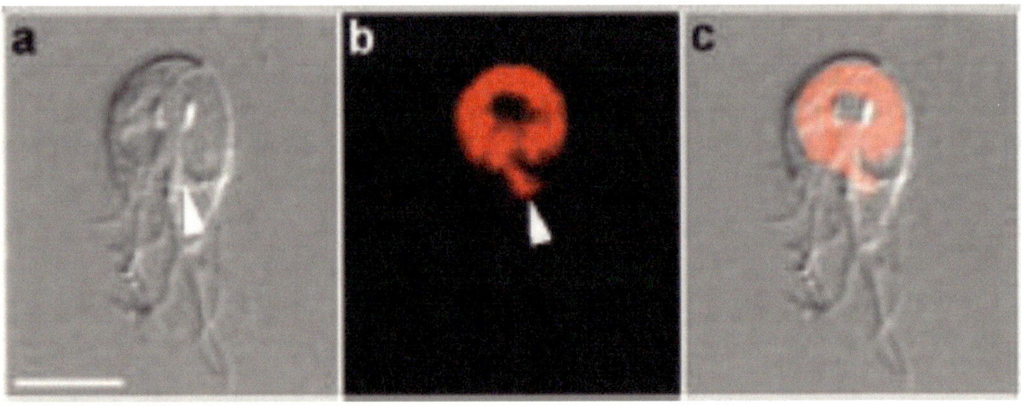

Figure 8. Immunofluorescence localization of β-giardin in *Giardia*, using the monoclonal antibody 7G9. The disk presents positive labeling as well the MB (arrowheads). (a) DIC visualization; (b) immunofluorescence; (c) overlay [74]. Bar = 5 μm.

out in the direction of the v rods associated with the lateral-posterior flagella (**Figure 9a–d**). Bridges of different lengths interconnect the *funis* microtubules [78] (**Figure 9a–d**). The microtubular sheets of this structure are covered by a lattice-like array of unidentified material, as revealed by HIM analysis [18]. In a previous work, an actin helix was shown to bundle the axonemes of the caudal flagella. In the final portion of the caudal complex, an association of the microtubules with cytoplasmic filaments was found [27]. It is proposed that the funis, together with the other axonemes, could work as a flexible cord and be responsible for the caudal movement of the cells such as lateral bending and dorsal-ventral flexion [70, 78; see Section 2.2.3].

2.5. Filament network

It has been shown that *G. intestinalis* genome contains a single divergent actin gene with an identity that is 58% similar to actin from other cells [79]. In addition, no genes coding for actin-binding proteins, formin, and myosin were found [11]. Further characterization of the *Giardia* actin showed that it is localized in several regions of the cell (cortex, axonemes, nuclei) and polymerizes *in vitro*, forming true microfilaments [27]. Some authors observed that drugs, which interfere with actin dynamic such as cytochalasin D and jasplakinolide, inhibited cytokinesis, and induced fragmentation of ventral disk and ventro-lateral flange [70, 80, 81]. Knockdown of the *Giardia* actin gene (giActin) interferes with clathrin-mediated endocytosis, membrane trafficking of CWP, and cytokinesis [27]. Subsequently, it was

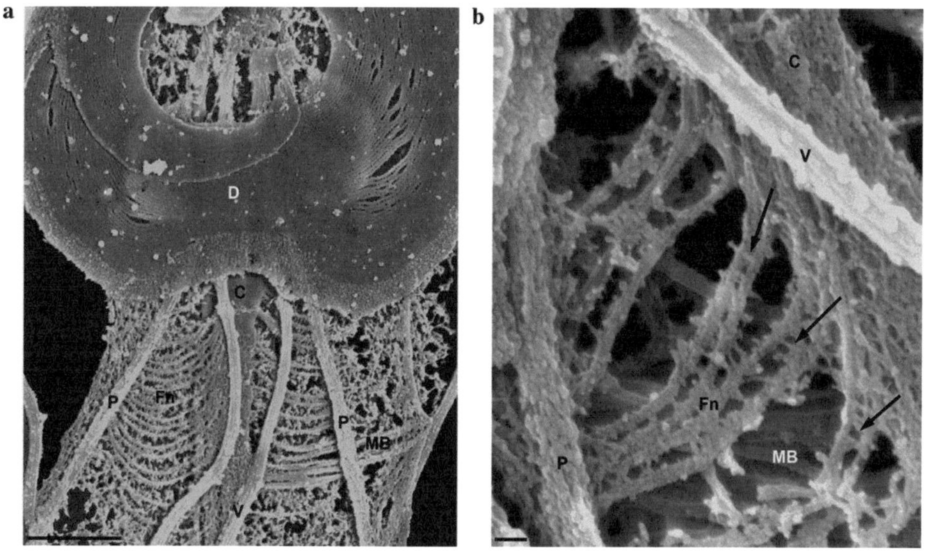

Figure 9. SEM of *G. intestinalis* in a ventral view. (a) Note that the microtubules of the *funis* (Fn) emanate from the caudal flagella (C) and are anchored to the posterior-lateral flagella (P). The median body (MB) is also appears as bundles of microtubules close to the *funis*. The arrows point to nuclei prints which are located dorsally to the ventral disk (D). (b) FESEM of *G. intestinalis* in a close view. The *funis* microtubules (Fn) are observed emanating from the caudal flagella (C) toward the posterior-lateral flagella (P). Notice that the microtubules present links (arrows), many of which were disrupted by the extraction treatment. The median body (MB), also formed by microtubules, is seen in a dorsal position in relation to the *funis*. Ventral flagella (V) [78]. Bar = 1 μm (a) and 100 nm (b).

shown that *Giardia* contains around 80 putative actin-binding proteins that may constitute a set of evolutionarily indispensable, actin-interacting proteins [82]. Using immunofluorescence approaches with specific antibodies combined with 3D-structured illumination light microscopy, Paredez et al. [27] showed that *Giardia* actin could form C-shaped filaments and helix-structures. A looser meshwork of filaments with a mean diameter of 9 nm was recently observed in the cytoskeleton of *G. intestinalis* using HIM [18]. The filaments spread out along the dorsal region and formed ring array structures [18] (**Figure 10a, b**). Immunogold labeling associated with UHRSEM coupled to backscattered electron detectors showed a labeling for actin in this region. These filaments therefore may correspond to microfilaments, which could act as a scaffold and provide support for the dorsal surface and cellular components [18]. Interestingly, Weiland et al. [59] observed that *Giardia* present several annexins, which are proteins known to interact with the F-actin in other cell models. Because annexins are associated with the trophozoite membrane, the Weiland team suggested that annexins could stabilize the cytoskeleton by cross-linking the plasma membrane to the underlying microtubules/microfilaments.

2.6. Behavior of the cytoskeleton during differentiation and cell division

The differentiation of trophozoites into cysts is an important process that allows the survival of the parasite under stress conditions of the environmental milieu. Morphological analyses using scanning and transmission electron microscopy show that during trophozoite-cyst transformation, several modifications occur [68, 83, 84]. Midlej and Benchimol [68] showed that in the early stages of encystment, the trophozoite gradually changes from its flattened form to an oval/rounded shape. This is accomplished by an increase in the membranous structure of the flange, which curves, causing cell folding and the formation

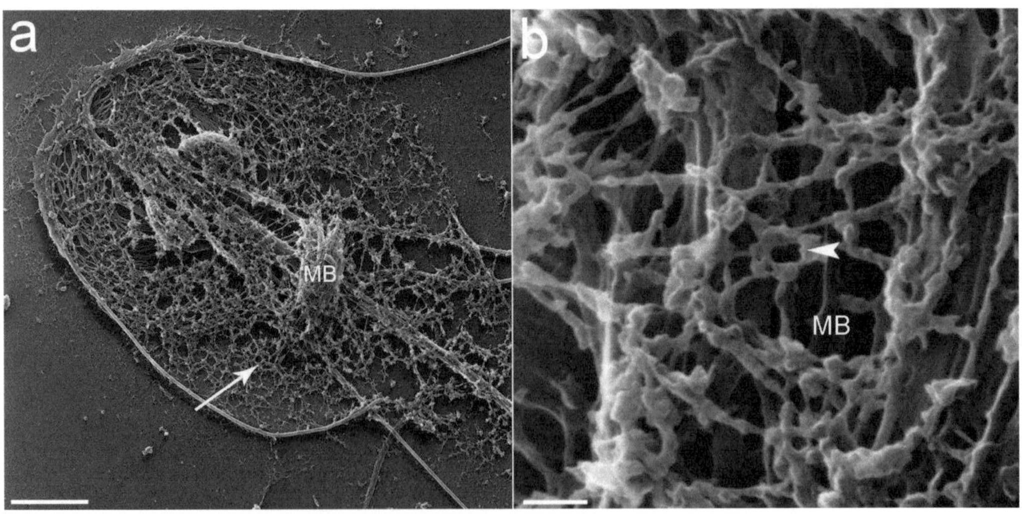

Figure 10. Dorsal view of Giardia by HIM. (a) Cytoplasmic filaments (arrow) contacting cytoskeletal structures such as the median body (MB). (b) High magnification of (a). It is possible to observe a ring array (arrowhead) [18]. Bars: 2 μm (a); 100 nm (b).

of the concave depression in the ventral region. In addition, the fibrillar material is deposited gradually on the encysting cells forming the cystic wall. At the same time, alterations also occur in the ventral disk spiral, which opens up and then assumed a horse-shaped structure. In the later stages of encystment, this structure fragments into four parts. These authors also observed that during differentiation of the trophozoite-cyst, the flagella are gradually internalized and kept in vacuoles. The ventral flagella are enclosed firstly by folding of the flange membrane. The last flagella to be internalized are the caudal that form a tail that persists until the last stages of the process. The flagella beating are still observed inside the cell. Midlej and Benchimol [68] demonstrated also the presence of an operculum in the final stage of the encystment, before the complete closing of the cyst. They suggested that this opening could be a weak region of the cyst, which would facilitate the exit of the trophozoite observed during encystment. During differentiation of the cyst into trophozoites, the flagella protrude through a small opening in the cyst wall, which is enlarged by flagella motion. The trophozoites emerged from cyst are oval in shape and quickly become flattened and elongate [71, 85].

The reorganization of the *Giardia* cytoskeleton also occurs during cell division [58]. Sagolla et al. demonstrated that *Giardi*a has a semi-open mitosis with two extranuclear spindles responsible for chromosome segregation. Using time-lapsed, confocal, and electron microscopy, Tumová et al. [72] described the different steps of *Giardia* cell division. According to these authors, the division begins in adhered cells by the detachment of the microtubule of the ventral disk from basal bodies. The overlapping region of the disk loosens and the central bare area increases. These alterations are accomplished by shortening and subsequent disappearance of the microribbons. At end of this stage, the nuclei are duplicated.

The rearrangement of the flagellar axonemes seems to take place in prophase when nuclear migration occurs in the cell midline [58]. Using light and electron microscopy and immunofluorescence methods, Nohýnková et al. [56] demonstrated that *Giardia* reorganize the flagellar apparatus during semi-conservative cell division. Each daughter *Giardia* receives four flagella from the parent cell, while the other flagella are assembled *de novo* in each cell. During this process, basal bodies/flagella migrate, assume different positions, and transform to different flagellar types in progeny until their maturation is completed [56]. As observed by Tumová et al. [72], after reorientation of the anterior flagella, the daughter cell disks are organized on the anterior dorsal side and positioned laterally. During this phase, lateral crest and ventro-lateral flange are not visualized. The Tumová team observed that in the final steps of cell division, the trophozoites are seen joined by their posterior region and swim freely in the medium, while the new disks are assembled. The daughter cells with fully developed disks (i.e., with the presence of lateral crest and flange) attach to a substrate but are still connected tail to tail by a cytoplasmic bridge. The cell division ends by a process resembling adhesion-dependent cytokinesis. Although these authors have suggested that the splitting of the diving organism occurs in ventral-ventral axial symmetry in the plane of the daughter disks, previous studies show that other types of cytokinesis (dorsal-dorsal or ventral-dorsal axial symmetry) may occur in *Giardia* [86].

Author details

Ana Paula Rocha Gadelha[1], Marlene Benchimol[2] and Wanderley de Souza[3*]

*Address all correspondence to: wsouza@biof.ufrj.br

1 National Institute of Metrology, Quality and Technology, Rio de Janeiro, Brasil

2 Biophisics Institute - Federal University of Rio de Janeiro, Rio de Janeiro, Brasil

3 CENABIO - National Center for Structural Biology and Bioimaging and National Institute of Science and Technology on Structural Biology and Bioimaging, Rio de Janeiro, Brasil

References

[1] Buret AG. Pathophysiology of enteric infections with *Giardia duodenalis*. Parasite. 2008;**15**:261-265. DOI: 10.1051/parasite/2008153261

[2] Karanis P, Kourenti C, Smith H. Waterborne transmission of protozoan parasites: A worldwide review of outbreaks and lessons learnt. Journal of Water and Health. 2007;**5**:1-38

[3] Adam RD. Biology of *Giardia lamblia*. Clinical Microbiology Reviews. 2001;**14**:447-475. DOI: 10.1128/CMR.14.3.447-475.2001

[4] Bingham AK, Meyer EA. *Giardia* excystation can be induced *in vitro* in acidic solution. Nature. 1979;**227**:301-302

[5] Boucher SE, Gillin FD. Excystation of in vitro-derived *Giardia lamblia* cysts. Infection and Immunity. 1990;**58**:3516-3522

[6] Ankarklev J, Jerlström-Hultqvist J, Ringqvist E, Troell K, Svärd SG. Behind the smile: Cell biology and disease mechanisms of *Giardia* species. Nature Reviews Microbiology. 2010;**8**:413-422. DOI: 10.1038/nrmicro2317

[7] Halliez MC, Buret AG. Extra-intestinal and long term consequences of *Giardia duodenalis* infections. World Journal of Gastroenterology. 2013;**19**:8974-8985. DOI: 10.3748/wjg.v19.i47.8974

[8] Teoh DA, Kamieeniecki D, Pang G, Buret AG. *Giardia lamblia* rearranges F-actin and alpha-actinin in human colonic and duodenal monolayers and reduces transepithelial electrical resistance. Journal of Parasitology. 2000;**86**:800-806. DOI: 10.1645/00223395(2000)086[0800:GLRFAA]2.0.CO;2

[9] Scott KG, Meddings JB, Kirk DR, Lees-Miller SP, Buret AG. Intestinal infection with *Giardia* spp. reduces epithelial barrier function in a myosin light chain kinase-dependent fashion. Gastroenterology. 2002;**123**:1179-1190

[10] Maia-Brigagão C, Morgado-Díaz JA, de Souza W. *Giardia* disrupts the arrangement of tight, adherens and desmosomal junction proteins of intestinal cells. Parasitology International. 2012;**61**:280-287. DOI: 10.1016/j.parint.2011.11.002

[11] Elmendorf HG, Dawson SC, McCaffery JM. The cytoskeleton of *Giardia lamblia*. International Journal of Parasitology. 2003;**33**:3-28

[12] Cheissin EM. Ultrastructure of *L. duodenalis*. I. Body surface, sucking disk and median bodies. Journal of Protozoology. 1964;**11**:19-98

[13] Holberton DV. Fine structure of the ventral disc apparatus and the mechanism of attachment in the flagellate *Giardia muris*. Journal of Cell Science. 1973;**13**:11-41

[14] Brown JR, Schwartz CL, Heumann JM, Dawson SC, Hoenger A. A detailed look at the cytoskeletal architecture of the *Giardia lamblia* ventral disc. Journal of Structural Biology. 2016;**194**:38-48. DOI: 10.1016/j.jsb.2016.01.01

[15] Campanati L, de Souza W. The cytoskeleton of *Giardia lamblia*. Trends in Cell & Molecular Biology. 2009;**4**:49-61

[16] Schwartz CL, Heumann JM, Dawson SC, Hoenger A. A detailed, hierarchical study of *Giardia lamblia*'s ventral disc reveals novel microtubule-associated protein complexes. PLoS One. 2012;**7**:e43783. DOI: 10.1371/journal.pone.0043783

[17] Crossley R, Marshall J, Clark JT, Holberton DV. Immunocytochemical differentiation of microtubules in the cytoskeleton of *Giardia lamblia* using monoclonal antibodies to alpha-tubulin and polyclonal antibodies to associated low molecular weight proteins. Journal of Cell Science. 1986;**180**:233-252

[18] Gadelha AP, Benchimol M, de Souza W. Helium ion microscopy and ultra-high-resolution scanning electron microscopy analysis of membrane-extracted cells reveals novel characteristics of the cytoskeleton of *Giardia intestinalis*. Journal of Structural Biology. 2015;**190**:271-278

[19] Kattenbach WM, Pimenta PF, de Souza W, Pinto da Silva P. *Giardia duodenalis*: A freeze-fracture, fracture-flip and cytochemistry study. Parasitology Research. 1991;**77**:651-658

[20] Lanfredi-Rangel A, Diniz JA, de Souza W. Presence of a protrusion on the ventral disk of adhered trophozoites of *Giardia lamblia*. Parasitology Research. 1999;**85**:951-955

[21] Campanati L, Sant'Anna C, Gadelha C, Lourenço D, Labati-Terra L, Bittencourt-Silvestre J, Benchimol M, Cunha-e-Silva NL, De Souza W. Improvement on the visualization of cytoskeletal structures of protozoan parasites using high-resolution field emission scanning electron microscopy (FESEM). Histochemistry and Cell Biology. 2005;**124**:87-95. DOI: 10.1007/s00418-005-0786-1

[22] Feely DE, Erlandsen SL, Chase DG, Holberton DV, Erlandsen SL. The biology of *Giardia*. In: Meyer EA, editor. Giardiasis. New York: Elsevier; 1990. pp. 11-49

[23] Holberton DV, Ward AP. Isolation of the cytoskeleton from *Giardia*: tubulin and a low-molecular-weight protein associated with microribbon structure. Journal of Cell Science. 1981;**47**:139-166

[24] Chavez B, Martinez-Palomo A. *Giardia lamblia*: Freeze-fracture ultrastructure of the ventral disc plasma membrane. Journal of Eukaryotic Microbiology. 1995;**42**:136-141

[25] Feely DE, Schollmeyer JV, Erlandsen SL. *Giardia spp*: Distribution of contractile proteins in the attachment organelle. Experimental Parasitology. 1982;**53**:145-154

[26] Hagen KD, Hirakawa MP, House SA, Schwartz CL, Pham JK, Cipriano MJ, De La Torre MJ, Sek AC, Du G, Forsythe BM, Dawson SC. Novel structural components of the ventral disc and lateral crest in *Giardia intestinalis*. PLoS Neglected Tropical Diseases. 2011;**5**:e1442. DOI: 10.1371/journal.pntd.0001442

[27] Paredez AR, Assaf ZJ, Sept D, Timofejeva L, Dawson SC, Wang CJ, Cande WZ. An actin cytoskeleton with evolutionarily conserved functions in the absence of canonical actin-binding proteins. Proceedings of the National Academy of Sciences of the United States of America. 2011;**108**:6151-6156. DOI: 10.1073/pnas.1018593108

[28] Kirk-Mason KE, Turner MJ, Chakraborty PR. Cloning and sequence of beta tubulin cDNA from *Giardia lamblia*. Nucleic Acids Research. 1988;**16**:2733

[29] Kirk-Mason KE, Turner MJ, Chakraborty PR. Evidence for unusually short tubulin mRNA leaders and characterization of tubulin genes in *Giardia lamblia*. Molecular and Biochemical Parasitology. 1989;**36**:87-99

[30] Soltys BJ, Gupta RS. Immunoelectron microscopy of *Giardia lamblia* cytoskeleton using antibody to acetylated alpha-tubulin. Journal of Eukaryotic Microbiology. 1994;**41**:625-632

[31] Weber K, Schneider A, Westermann S, Muller N, Plessmann U. Posttranslational modifications of alpha-and beta-tubulin in *Giardia lamblia*, an ancient eukaryote. FEBS Letters. 1997;**419**:87-91

[32] Campanati L, Bré MH, Levilliers N, de Souza W. Expression of tubulin polyglycylation in *Giardia lamblia*. Biology of the Cell. 1999;**91**:499-506

[33] Campanati L, Troester H, Monteiro-Leal LH, Spring H, Trendelenburg MF, de Souza W. Tubulin diversity in trophozoites of *Giardia lamblia*. Histochemistry and Cell Biology. 2003;**119**:323-331. DOI: 10.1007/s00418-003-0517-4

[34] Crossley R, Holberton D. Assembly of 2.5 nm filaments from giardin, a protein associated with cytoskeletal microtubules in *Giardia*. Journal of Cell Science. 1985;**78**:205-231

[35] Morgan RO, Fernandez MP. Molecular phylogeny of annexins and identification of a primitive homologue in *Giardia lamblia*. Molecular Biology and Evolution. 1995;**12**:967-979

[36] Bauer B, Engelbrecht S, Bakker-Grunwald T, Scholze H. Functional identification of alpha 1-giardin as an annexin of *Giardia lamblia*. FEMS Microbiology Letters. 1999;**173**:147-153

[37] Weeratunga SK, Osman A, Hu NJ, Wang CK, Mason L, Svärd S, Hope G, Jones MK, Hofmann A. Alpha-1 giardin is an annexin with highly unusual calcium-regulated mechanisms. Journal of Molecular Biology. 2012;**423**:169-181

[38] Weber K, Geisler N, Plessmann U, Bremerich A, Lechtreck KF, Melkonian M. SF-assemblin, the structural protein of the 2-nm filaments from striated microtubule associated fibers of algal flagellar roots, forms a segmented coiled coil. Journal of Cell Science. 1993;**12**:837-845

[39] Macarisin D, O'Brien C, Fayer R, Bauchan G, Jenkins M. Immunolocalization of β-and δ-giardin within the ventral disk in trophozoites of *Giardia duodenalis* using multiplex laser scanning confocal microscopy. Parasitology Research. 2012;**111**:241-248. DOI: 10.1016/j.jmb.2012.06.041

[40] Palm JE, Weiland ME, Griffiths WJ, Ljungström I, Svärd SG. Identification of immunoreactive proteins during acute human giardiasis. Journal of Infectious Diseases. 2003;**187**:1849-1859. DOI: 10.1086/375356

[41] Lourenço D, Andrade IS, Terra LL, Guimarães PR, Zingali RB, de Souza W. Proteomic analysis of the ventral disc of *Giardia lamblia*. BMC Research Notes. 2012 Jan 19;**5**:41. DOI: 10.1186/1756-0500-5-41

[42] Holberton DV. Attachment of *Giardia*: hydrodynamic model based on flagellar activity. Journal of Experimental Biology. 1974;**60**:207-221

[43] Erlandsen SL, Russo AP, Turner JN. Evidence for adhesive activity of the ventrolateral flange in *Giardia lamblia*. Journal of Eukaryotic Microbiology. 2004;**51**:73-80

[44] Lenaghan SC, Davis CA, Henson WR, Zhang Z, Zhang M. High-speed microscopic imaging of flagella motility and swimming in *Giardia lamblia* trophozoites. Proceedings of the National Academy of Sciences of the United States of America. 2011;**108**:E550-E558. DOI: 10.1073/pnas.1106904108

[45] Campanati L, Holloschi A, Troster H, Spring H, de Souza W, Monteiro-Leal LH. Video-microscopy observations of fast dynamic processes in the protozoon *Giardia lamblia*. Cell Motility and the Cytoskeleton. 2002;**51**:213-224. DOI: 10.1002/cm.10026

[46] House SA, Richter DJ, Pham JK, Dawson SC. *Giardia* flagellar motility is not directly required to maintain attachment to surfaces. PLoS Pathogens. 2011;**7**:e1002167. DOI: 10.1371/journal.ppat.1002167

[47] Woessner DJ, Dawson SC. The *Giardia* median body protein is a ventral disc protein that is critical for maintaining a domed disc conformation during attachment. Eukaryotic Cell. 2012;**11**:292-301. DOI: 10.1128/EC.05262-11

[48] Pegado MG, de Souza W. Role of surface components in the interaction of process of *Giardia duodenalis* with epithelial cells in vitro. Parasitology Research. 1994;**80**:320-326

[49] Magne D, Favennce L, Chochillon C, Gorenflot A, Meillet D, Kapel N, Raichvarg D, Savel J, Gobert JG. Role of cytoskeleton and surface lectins in *Giardia duodenalis* attachament to Caco 2 cells. Parasitology Research. 1991;**77**:659-662

[50] Katelaris PH, Naeem A, Farthing MJ. Attachment of *Giardia lamblia* trophozoites to a cultured human intestinal cell line. Gut. 1995;**37**:512-518

[51] Benchimol M. Participation of the adhesive disc during karyokinesis in *Giardia lamblia*. Biology of the Cell. 2004;**96**:291-301. DOI: 10.1016/j.biolcel.2004.01.007

[52] Maia-Brigagão C, Gadelha AP, de Souza W. New associated structures of the anterior flagella of *Giardia duodenalis*. Microscopy and Microanalysis. 2013;**19**:1374-1376. DOI: 10.1017/S1431927613013275

[53] Friend DS. The fine structure of *Giardia muris*. Journal of Cell Biology. 1966;**29**:317-332

[54] de Souza W, Campanati L, Attias M. Strategies and results of field emission scanning electron microscopy (FE-SEM) in the study of parasitic protozoa. Micron. 2008;**39**:77-87

[55] Kulda J, Nohýnková E. Flagellates of the human intestine and of intestines of other species. In: Kreier JP, editor. Parasitic Protozoa. New York: Academic Press; 1978. pp. 69-138

[56] Nohynková E, Tumová P, Kulda J. Cell division of *Giardia intestinalis*: Flagellar developmental cycle involves transformation and exchange of flagella between mastigonts of a diplomonad cell. Eukaryotic Cell. 2006;**5**:753-761. DOI: 10.1128/EC.5.4.753-761.2006

[57] McInally SG, Dawson SC. Eight unique basal bodies in the multi-flagellated diplomonad *Giardia lamblia*. Cilia. 2016; **4**:5-21. DOI: 10.1186/s13630-016-0042-4

[58] Sagolla MS, Dawson SC, Mancuso JJ, Cande WZ. Three-dimensional analysis of mitosis and cytokinesis in the binucleate parasite *Giardia intestinalis*. Journal of Cell Science. 2006;**119**:4889-4900. DOI: 10.1242/jcs.03276

[59] Weiland ME, McArthur AG, Morrison HG, Sogin ML, Svärd SG. Annexin-like alpha giardins: A new cytoskeletal gene family in *Giardia lamblia*. International Journal for Parasitology. 2005;**35**:617-626. DOI: 10.1016/j.ijpara.2004.12.009

[60] Steuart RF, O'Handley R, Lipscombe RJ, Lock RA, Thompson RC. Alpha 2 giardin is an assemblage A-specific protein of human infective *Giardia duodenalis*. Parasitology. 2008;**135**:1621-1627. DOI: 10.1017/S0031182008004988

[61] Vahrmann A, Sarić M, Koebsch I, Scholze H. Alpha14-Giardin (annexin E1) is associated with tubulin in trophozoites of *Giardia lamblia* and forms local slubs in the flagella. Parasitology Research. 2008;**102**:321-326. DOI: 10.1007/s00436-007-0758-6

[62] Pathuri P, Nguyen ET, Ozorowski G, Svärd SG, Luecke H. Apo and calcium-bound crystal structures of cytoskeletal protein alpha-14 giardin (annexin E1) from the intestinal protozoan parasite *Giardia lamblia*. Journal of Molecular Biology. 2009;**385**:1098-1112. DOI: 10.1016/j.jmb.2008.11.012

[63] Elmendorf HG, Rohrer SC, Khoury RS, Bouttenot RE, Nash TE. Examination of a novel head-stalk protein family in *Giardia lamblia* characterised by the pairing of ankyrin repeats and coiled-coil domains. International Journal of Parasitology. 2005;**35**:1001-1011. DOI: 10.1016/j.ijpara.2005.03.009

[64] Hoeng JC, Dawson SC, House SA, Sagolla MS, Pham JK, Mancuso JJ, Löwe J, Cande WZ. High-resolution crystal structure and *in vivo* function of a kinesin-2 homologue in *Giardia intestinalis*. Molecular Biology of the Cell. 2008;**19**:3124-3137. DOI: 10.1091/mbc.E07-11-1156

[65] Nohýnkova E, Dráber P, Reischig J, Kulda J. Localization of gamma-tubulin in interphase and mitotic cells of a unicellular eukaryote *Giardia intestinalis*. European Journal of Cell Biology. 2000;**79**:438-445. DOI: 10.1078/0171-9335-00066

[66] Corrêa G, Morgado-Diaz JA, Benchimol M. Centrin in *Giardia lamblia*–ultrastructural localization. FEMS Microbiology Letters. 2004;**233**:91-96. DOI: 10.1016/j.femsle.2004.01.043

[67] Lauwaet T, Smith AJ, Reiner DS, Romijn EP, Wong CC, Davids BJ, Shah SA, Yates JR, Gillin FD. Mining the *Giardia* genome and proteome for conserved and unique basal body proteins. International Journal for Parasitology. 2011;**41**:1079-1092. DOI: 10.1016/j.ijpara.2011.06.001

[68] Midlej V, Benchimol M. *Giardia lamblia* behavior during encystment: How morphological changes in shape occur. Parasitology International. 2009;**58**:72-80. DOI: 10.1016/j.parint.2008.11.002

[69] Ghosh S, Frisardi M, Rogers R, Samuelson J. How *Giardia* swim and divide. Infection and Immunity. 2001;**69**:7866-7872. DOI: 10.1128/IAI.69.12.7866-7872.2001

[70] Carvalho KP, Monteiro-Leal LH. The caudal complex of *Giardia lamblia* and its relation to motility. Experimental Parasitology. 2004;**108**:154-162. DOI: 10.1016/j.exppara.2004.08.007

[71] Coggins JR, Schaefer FW. *Giardia muris:* Scanning electron microscopy of *in vitro* excystation. Experimental Parasitology. 1984;**57**:62-67

[72] Tumova P, Kulda J, Nohynkova E. Cell division of *Giardia intestinalis*: Assembly and disassembly of the adhesive disc and the cytokinesis. Cell Motility and Cytoskeleton. 2007;**64**:288-298. DOI: 10.1002/cm.20183

[73] Nosala C, Dawson SC. The critical role of the cytoskeleton in the pathogenesis of *Giardia*. Current Clinical Microbiology Reports. 2015;**2**:155-162. DOI: 10.1007/s40588-015-0026-y

[74] Piva B, Benchimol M. The median body of *Giardia lamblia*: An ultrastructural study. Biology of the Cell. 2004;**96**:735-746. DOI: 10.1016/j.biolcel.2004.05.006

[75] Brugerolle G. Contribuition a l'etude cytologique e phyletique des diplozoaires (Zoomastigophorea, Diplozoa Dangeard 1910). V. Nouvelle interpretation de l'organisation cellulaire de *Giardia*. Protistologica. 1975;**11**:99-109

[76] Meng TC, Aley SB, Svard SG, Smith MW, Huang B, Kim J, Gillin FD. Immunolocalization and sequence of caltractin/centrin from the early branching eukaryote *Giardia lamblia*. Molecular and Biochemical Parasitology. 1996;**79**:103-108

[77] Dawson SC, Sagolla MS, Mancuso JJ, Woessner DJ, House SA, Fritz-Laylin L, Cande WZ. Kinesin-13 regulates flagellar, interphase, and mitotic microtubule dynamics in *Giardia intestinalis*. Eukaryotic Cell. 2007;**6**:2354-2364. DOI: 10.1128/EC.00128-07

[78] Benchimol M, Piva B, Campanati L, de Souza W. Visualization of the funis of *Giardia lamblia* by high-resolution field emission scanning electron microscopy–New insights. Journal of Structural Biology. 2004;**147**:102-115. DOI: 10.1016/j.jsb.2004.01.017

[79] Morrison HG, McArthur AG, Gillin FD, Aley SB, Adam RD, Olsen GJ, Best AA, Cande WZ, Chen F, Cipriano MJ, Davids BJ, Dawson SC, Elmendorf HG, Hehl AB, Holder ME, Huse SM, Kim UU, Lasek-Nesselquist E, Manning G, Nigam A, Nixon JE, Palm D, Passamaneck NE, Prabhu A, Reich CI, Reiner DS, Samuelson J, Svard SG, Sogin ML. Genomic minimalism in the early diverging intestinal parasite *Giardia lamblia*. Science. 2007;**317**:1921-1926. DOI: 10.1126/science.1143837

[80] Corrêa G, Benchimol M. *Giardia lamblia* behavior under cytochalasins treatment. Parasitology Research. 2006;**98**:250-256. DOI: 10.1007/s00436-005-0065-z

[81] Castillo-Romero A, Leon-Avila G, Perez Rangel A, Cortes Zarate R, Garcia Tovar C, Hernandez JM. Participation of actin on *Giardia lamblia* growth and encystation. PLoS One. 2009;**4**:e7156. DOI: 10.1371/journal.pone.0007156

[82] Paredez AR, Nayeri A, Xu JW, Krtková J, Cande WZ. Identification of obscure yet conserved actin-associated proteins in *Giardia lamblia*. Eukaryotic Cell. 2014;**13**:776-784. DOI: 10.1128/EC.00041-14

[83] Benchimol M. The release of secretory vesicle in encysting *Giardia lamblia*. FEMS Microbiology Letters. 2004;**235**:81-87. DOI: 10.1016/j.femsle.2004.04.014

[84] Bittencourt-Silvestre J, Lemgruber L, de Souza W. Encystation process of *Giardia lamblia*: Morphological and regulatory aspects. Archives of Microbiology. 2010;**192**:259-265. DOI: 10.1007/s00203-010-0554-z

[85] Buchel LA, Gorenflot A, Chochillon C, Savel J, Gobert JG. *In vitro* excystation of *Giardia* from humans: A scanning electron microscopy study. Journal of Parasitology. 1987;**73**:487-493

[86] Benchimol M. Mitosis in *Giardia lamblia*: Multiple modes of cytokinesis. Protist. 2004;**155**: 33-44. DOI: 10.1078/1434461000162

Chapter 6

The Endomembrane System of *Giardia intestinalis*

Victor Midlej, Wanderley de Souza and
Marlene Benchimol

Additional information is available at the end of the chapter

http://dx.doi.org/10.5772/intechopen.70875

Abstract

Giardia intestinalis is a protozoan that colonizes the small intestine of virtually all mammals, adhering to the mucosal epithelial cells. It is a cosmopolitan parasite and agent of giardiasis, which can lead to human diarrheal diseases. The *Giardia* life cycle presents two forms—the trophozoite and the cyst—which are responsible for infection and transmission, respectively. This cell has been considered an excellent model for evolutionary studies, even though there are controversial hypotheses as to whether this parasite is an early eukaryote or not. *G. intestinalis* has a unique and very basic endomembrane system. The trophozoite gathers a very small pack of membrane-bounded structures: nuclei, endoplasmic reticulum (ER), peripheral vesicles (PV) and mitosomes. These organelles are involved in many functions from regulatory aspects in gene expression as well as membrane traffic events. Two functional nuclei are observed in the parasite; they are always located symmetrically in the anterior region of the trophozoite. The ER and PV commonly share and accumulate functions in the secretory pathway, they are responsible for endocytosis and digestion processes. The mitosome is a mitochondria-related organelle that does not produce ATP and lacks several mitochondrial characteristics. During the parasite differentiation into cyst, different types of vesicles appear into the cell body: the encystation specific vesicles (ESVs) and the encystation carbohydrate-positive vesicles (ECVs). These vesicles work together to form the parasite's cyst wall in order to ensure that the cell reaches the cyst stage. Interestingly, *Giardia* does not present a morphologically recognized Golgi apparatus. It has been claimed that during the encystation process, the ESVs could represent a Golgi-like structure, because this organelle presents some characteristics of that high eukaryotic Golgi apparatus. In this book chapter, we highlight the *G. intestinalis* endomembrane system, emphasizing their morphology, proteins involved in its organization as well as their functional role.

Keywords: parasite, morphology, giardiasis, ultrastructure

1. Introduction

1.1. *Giardia* and giardiasis

Giardia was observed for the first time by Antony Van Leeuwenhoek in 1681, but it was Lambl who described the cell morphological characteristics in detail and named it *Cercomonas intestinalis*. Subsequently, Blanchard changed the nomenclature in 1888 to *Giardia lamblia* [1–3]. The parasite is also known as *Giardia intestinalis, Giardia duodenalis, Giardia enterica* and *Lamblia intestinalis*. Currently, the preferred name is *G. intestinalis*.

The trophozoite of *G. intestinalis* inhabits the small intestine and causes the disease, whereas the cyst is protected by a cyst wall, can survive in adverse environmental conditions and thus is responsible for parasite transmission. Giardiasis starts when the cysts are ingested via food or contaminated water and reach the small intestine. The trophozoites emerge from the cyst wall and colonize the intestinal epithelium [4]. The emerged trophozoites adhere and spread out by binary divisions and form a monolayer over the intestinal mucosa provoking local inflammation and reduction in nutrient uptake. The parasites may reach the final portions of the intestine, becoming a cyst again, and they are liberated with the feces. The cysts can then infect new hosts [4]. Diarrhea is the main symptom of *G. intestinalis* infection, and giardiasis occurs in humans and several animals throughout the world. Giardial transmission between different species is frequent, and this characterizes giardiasis as a zoonotic disease [5]. The infection rates of giardiasis are associated with sanitary conditions since low rates are observed when sanitary conditions are implemented [6]. Giardiasis mainly affects children and is considered a cosmopolite disease [7]. Several factors such as geographic area, group of analysis, sensitivity of the diagnostic methods and health care accessibility influence the prevalence rates reported [8]. The disease treatment is based in nitroimidazole-derived drugs (metronidazole, tinidazole and ornidazole), since metronidazole is the most widely used drug [9].

2. Endomembrane system

The endomembrane system of higher eukaryotes comprises of a number of structures, such as the endoplasmic reticulum, nucleus, Golgi, lysosomes, peroxisomes, autophagosomes and vesicles involved in different traffic pathways. Many theories have addressed the evolutionary origin of eukaryotic membranes; the most acceptable one is the invagination of plasma membrane, which is based on the similarity between the endoplasmic reticulum (ER) lumen to the environment [10, 11].

Although *Giardia* belongs to the eukaryotic group, it lacks some of the typical organelles found in eukaryotes; therefore, this parasite is an interesting model to study cell evolution. Mitochondria and peroxisomes are not present in this parasite, as found in morphological and biochemical studies. In addition, Golgi complex and vesicles of the endocytic pathway are incipient. On the other hand, *Giardia* trophozoites exhibit membrane structures that incorporate the cationic, membrane potential-sensitive fluorophore rhodamine 123 and reduce a tetrazolium fluorogen. Based on this observation, the existence of membrane-associated sites with some similarities to

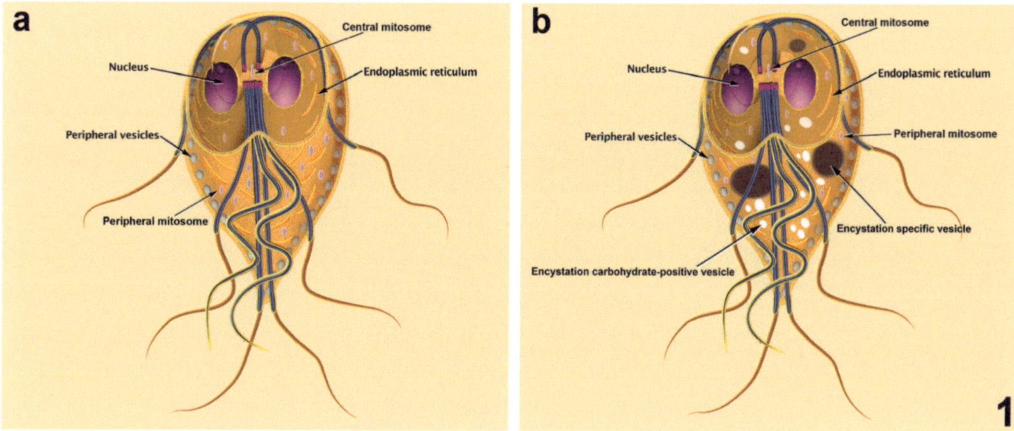

Figure 1. Endomembrane system of *G. intestinalis*. Schemes of a Giardia trophozoite (a) and when the process of encystation starts (b). Parasites present two nuclei. Both encystation vesicles ESV (encystation specific vesicle) and ECV (encystation carbohydrate-positive vesicle) are only present in the encysting cell. The ESVs are larger and dense, while the ECVs are smaller and lighter (b).

mitochondria has been suggested; an aerobic flagellate presenting mitochondria was proposed to possibly be the ancestor of *G. intestinalis* [12].

The membrane system of *G. intestinalis* comprises a unique set of vesicles named peripheral vesicles and a much diffused endoplasmic reticulum network. Moreover, this cell possesses two nuclei with a very similar nuclear membrane complex as observed in higher eukaryote cells (**Figure 1a**). During the differentiation of trophozoite to cysts, two types of membrane-bounded vesicles appear, the ESVs and ECVs, and both act to build the cyst wall, which is a constitutive and important structure of cyst (**Figure 1b**). Deeper in the encystation process, we face a paradigm: is there a Golgi-like structure in *Giardia*? Some authors claimed that during the encystation process, the ESVs assume some Golgi characteristics [13].

Below, we will discuss each of the membrane-bounded structures that compose the endomembrane system of *G. intestinalis* (**Figure 1**).

3. Peripheral vesicles

G. intestinalis belongs to the Giardiinae family, and it has a unique organellar system formed by numerous small vacuoles named peripheral vesicles (PVs) (**Figures 2–4**, **5c**, **9a**). The PVs are oval, elongated and are 100–200 nm in size (**Figure 2c**); they are located in the cell periphery, right below the plasma membrane (**Figure 2**) [14, 15]. The PVs have a fundamental role in the endocytosis process as well as during the digestion and retrograde transport of the parasite [16, 17]. A number of cytochemical studies indicated resident enzymes, such as acid phosphatases, sulfur-binding proteins (SH) and glucose-6-phosphatase in the PVs. The localization of these proteins pointed that the PVs present compatible functions to those initial or late

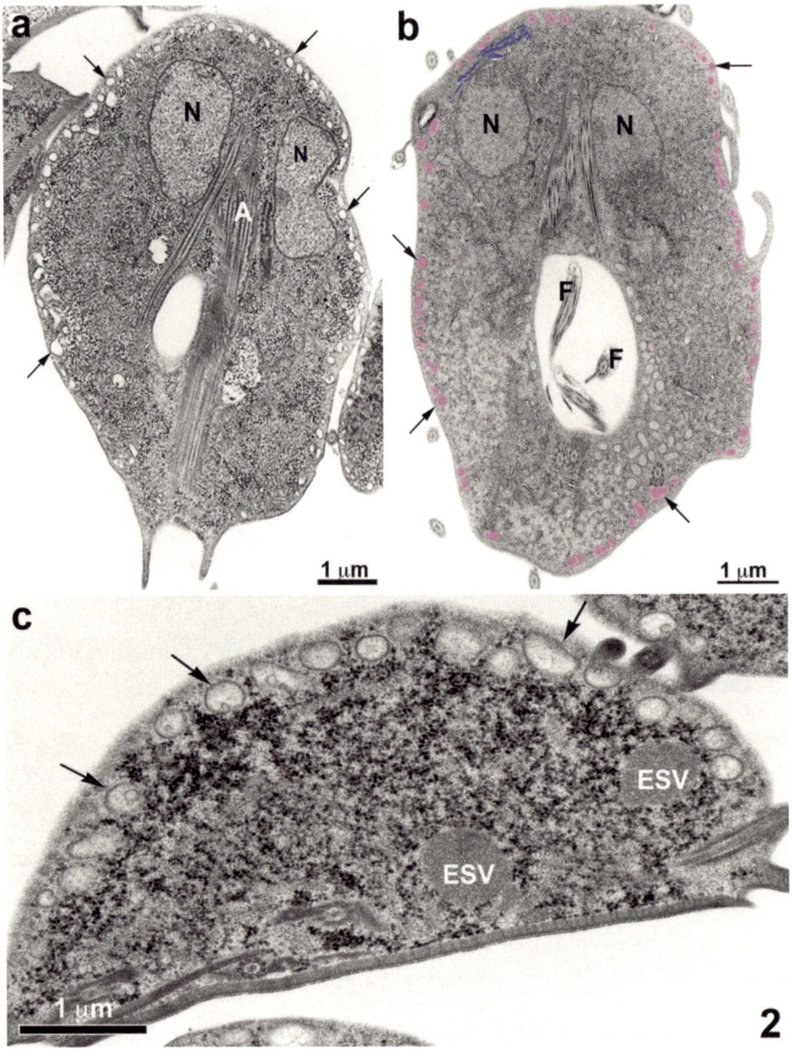

Figure 2. Peripheral vesicles of *G. intestinalis*. Transmission electron microscopy (TEM) of vegetative non-encysting (a and b) and encysting (c) parasite. The peripheral vesicles (PV, arrows) are right below the plasma membrane (a–c) and present similar size, shape and location in both forms (a–c). Artificially colored (b). N, nucleus; A, axoneme; F, flagellum; ESV, encystation-specific vesicle.

endosomes [17]. The accumulation of gold-labeled macromolecules such as albumin, peroxidase, transferrin and low-density lipoprotein in PVs [15] reinforced this idea. Moreover, the cytochemical localization of acid phosphatase, a classical lysosomal marker, in these vesicles Kattenbach and colleagues [15] led to the suggestion that *G. intestinalis* presents an endosomal-lysosomal system that later on during evolution was subdivided into compartments such as early or late endosomes and lysosomes [17]. Besides the degradation function played by the PVs, to date, it is the only known organelle involved in the *Giardia* endocytic pathway that is capable of accumulating fluid phase and membrane-bound molecules [18]. It was

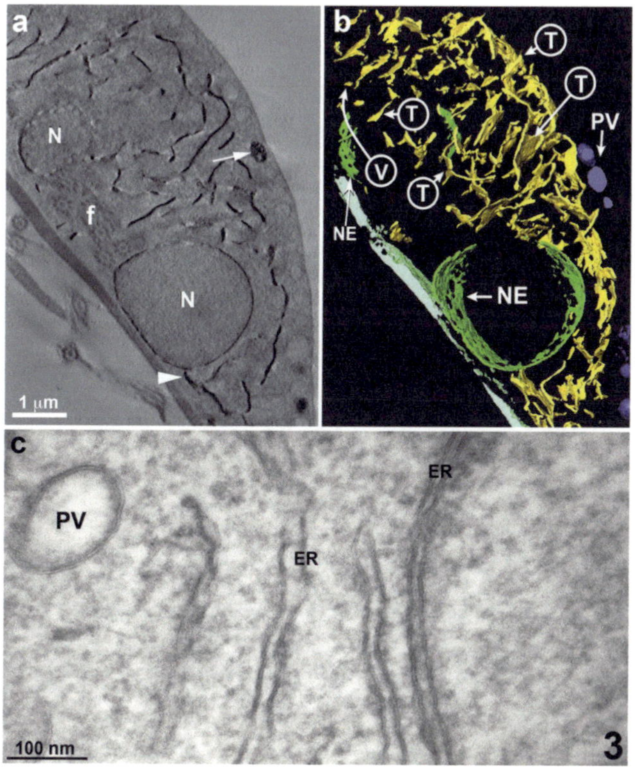

Figure 3. Endoplasmic reticulum of *G. intestinalis*. Electron tomography of a thick section after cytochemistry for glucose-6-phosphatase (a), 3-D reconstruction of the same cell (b) and TEM (c). (a) The reaction product is on the nuclear envelope (NE), the endoplasmic reticulum (ER) and some peripheral vesicles (PVs, arrow). An arrowhead indicates to a point near the ER and nuclear envelope (NE). (b). Distribution of ER tubules (T) (yellow) and cisternae (NE) (green) occupying the majority of space in the cytosol. PVs (blue). Cross section of the ER appears vesicular (V); ER longitudinal view: tubular (T). N, nucleus; f, flagella axonemes. (c) Note the ER profiles and its proximity to PVs. (figures a and b, from Abodeely et al. [19]); (figure c, unpublished).

demonstrated that these vesicles periodically open to the cell exterior either via a channel or by fusion with the plasma membrane and take up soluble material before closing again (**Figure 4**) [19]. The uptake of soluble material from the environment into PV is not selective, which is in contrast to further retrograde transport that allows only certain, yet undefined, substances to rapidly cross over into the proximal ER [19]. It has been demonstrated that three protein complexes are associated with the endocytic machinery in *Giardia*, showing a discrete localization in the cortical area of trophozoites by fluorescence microscopy [20, 21]. These protein complexes are the clathrin heavy chain (*Gl*CHC), subunits of the AP2 heterotetramer (*Gl*AP2) and Giardia dynamin-related protein (*Gl*DRP) [20, 21]. Recently, a detailed protein interactome of *Gl*CHC revealed all of the conserved factors in addition to a novel protein, a putative clathrin light chain [22]. However, there are no clathrin coated-vesicles in *Giardia*. It was claimed that the giardial clathrin is organized into static cores surrounded by dynamic interaction partners, which are most likely involved in the regulation of fusion between the plasma

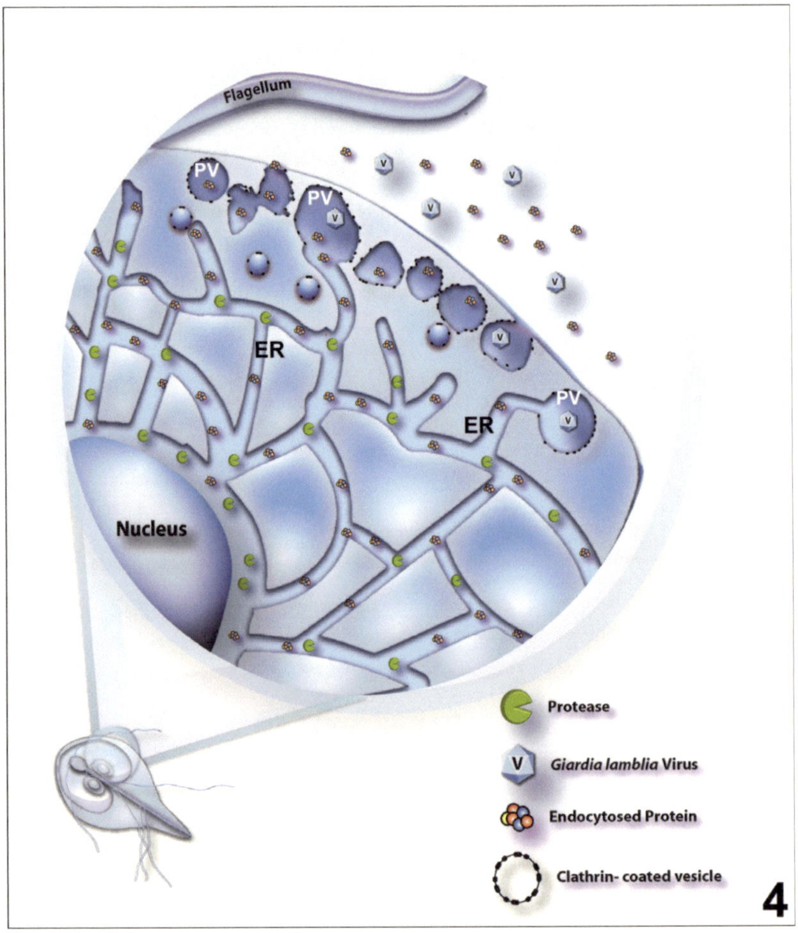

Figure 4. Schematic representation of the endocytic network of *G. intestinalis*. Active proteases reside primarily in the ER, where endocytosed proteins are degraded. PVs contain clathrin and are the site of initial uptake. Membrane fusions between PVs and between PVs and the ER are dynamic. Endocytosed proteins go from PVs to ER by dynamic fusions. ER, endoplasmic reticulum; PV, peripheral vesicles (from Abodeely et al. [19]).

membrane and the PVs in a "kiss-and-flush"-like mechanism [22]. These factors are key components of the clathrin-dependent endocytic machinery in higher eukaryotes and protozoa alike.

4. Endoplasmic reticulum

Although electron microscopy revealed similar structures to endoplasmic reticulum (ER), there is still a controversy concerning the real presence of this organelle in *Giardia*. The cloning and characterization of SRα, a receptor for signal recognition particle (SRP) as well as the use of binding immunoglobulin protein (BiP), a ER resident 70 kDa heat shock protein, allowed the identification of an extensive membrane system in *G. intestinalis* [23]. So far, the presence of an ER has been demonstrated in the parasite; moreover, three genes for protein disulfide isomerase (PDI) in *Giardia* were cloned and characterized, and its products were localized into ER [24]. Electron microscopy cytochemistry for glucose-6-phosphate, a resident ER enzyme, allowed the observation of an extensive reticular system in this parasite [17]. The ER presents a complex, bilaterally symmetrical organization that is distributed from the nuclear envelopes throughout the cell body (**Figure 3**). The presence of this archetypical eukaryotic organelle in *Giardia* has been called into question [16]. The ER in giardia trophozoites is composed by little tinny cisternae (**Figure 3c**), while during the encystation process, there is an increase in the ER cisternae number [17].

Although *G. intestinalis* has a conventional ER concerning the secretory trafficking, some elements are missing entirely, such as the post-translational modification machinery. The calnexin-calreticulin machinery, which acts in the quality control of N-glycosylated secreted proteins, is absent [25]. An extensive genomic and biochemical analyses demonstrated that the parasite lacks several nucleotide sugar transporters [26]. Thus, Asn-linked glycosylation in the giardial ER is limited to the addition of GlcNAc1–2 to proteins. A coordinated work among conserved machinery for translocation [27], and chaperones and members of the PDI family [28] support the co-translational import and folding of secreted proteins. Giardial PDIs play a major role in assisting the folding of the cyst wall proteins (CWPs) [29].

It was proposed that the *Giardia*'s reticulum would be a tubule-vesicular network with ER functions as well as endosomes and lysosomes activities by connections with the peripheral vesicles (**Figure 4**) [19]. Based on that, the ER of *G. intestinalis* possesses different functions (e.g., protein synthesis, endocytic activities and extracellular material degradation), since it is a pluripotent compartment [19].

5. Nuclear envelope

One of the most intriguing features of *G. intestinalis* trophozoite is the presence of two nuclei with mirror symmetry (**Figures 1**, **2a** and **b**, **5a**). The nuclei are spherical or oval and symmetrically placed in the anterior portion of the cell (**Figures 1**, **2a** and **b**, **8**). Both nuclei are equivalent; they have the same amount of chromosomes, 2n = 10, and show a great homology when the nucleotide sequences are compared [30].

An inner and an outer membrane compose the nuclear envelope of higher eukaryote cells. The outer membrane is continuous with the ER membrane, which presents ribosomes engaged in protein synthesis. The inner nuclear membrane contains, in addition to the trilaminar membrane, filamentous proteins that form the nuclear lamina, which provides structural support for this membrane. The nuclear envelope of all eukaryotes is perforated by elaborated structures known as nuclear pore complexes [31].

The *Giardia*'s nuclear envelope displays different profiles, such as blebs in the outer nuclear membrane envelope. This structure could correspond to the formation of vesicles from the endoplasmic reticulum that forms the outer nuclear membrane (**Figure 5**) [32]. Close proximity

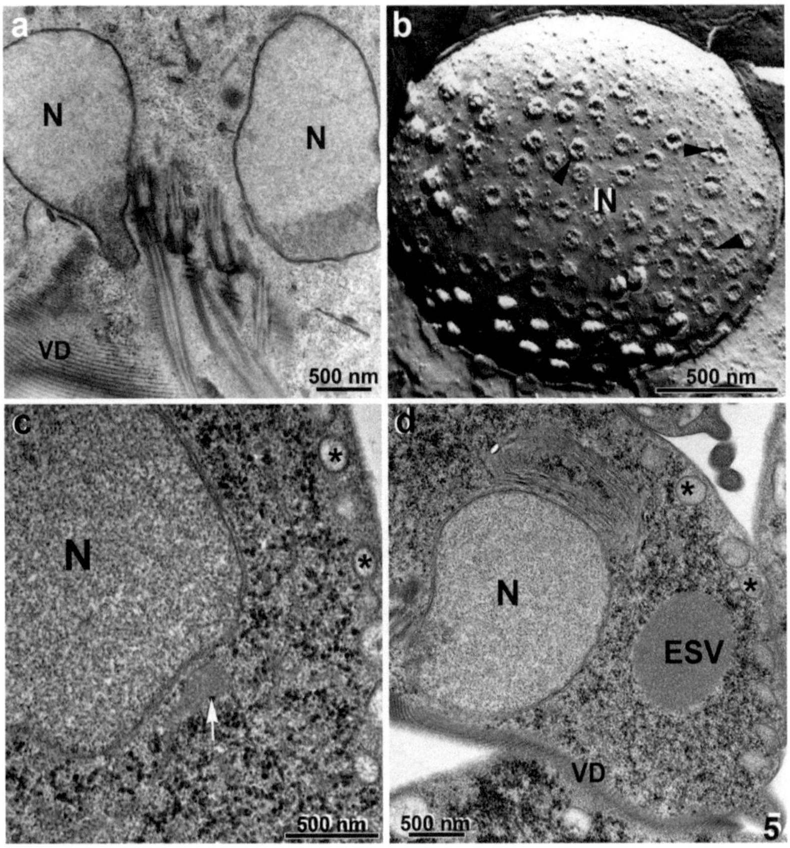

Figure 5. Nuclei of *G. intestinalis*. Transmission electron microscopy (a, c and d) and freeze-fractured (figure b) images in non-encysting cells (a and b) and under process of encystation (c and d). (a) Both nuclei are similar in size; basal bodies and axonemes are just between the nuclei. (b) Pore complexes (arrowheads) similar in size and shape, with annular substructures. (c) In early stages of encystation (10 h) a nascent ESV (arrow) is close to nuclear envelope. (d) After 21 h of encystation the ESVs are closer to the peripheral vesicles (asterisks) and plasma membrane. N, nuclei; VD, ventral disc; ESV, encystation specific vesicle. (figure a: from Benchimol [35]; figure b: from Benchimol [34]; figures c and d: Midlej V, De Souza W and Benchimol, unpublished).

areas exist between the two nuclear membranes that become parallel but are distinct from the diaphragms found in nuclear envelopes of the eukaryotic cells [33]. Interestingly, the parasite pore complex distribution and clustering is different in each nucleus. *Giardia* nuclei are not identical; they seem to be either in different phases of chromosome condensation or they have different metabolic activity. Dividing nuclei displayed very few pore complexes, which is a characteristic of low metabolic activity and/or low nucleus-cytoplasm transport. The pore complexes in *G. intestinalis* are very uniform in size and shape, and they contain annular substructures (**Figure 5b**) that are similar to those of higher eukaryotic cells [33].

The parasite mitosis is not similar to other organisms, presenting different characteristics: (1) the nuclear envelope does not fragment completely during mitosis, leaving open places on the nuclei poles. This type of division is named semi-open mitosis, because only the nuclear poles are open. The spindle microtubules penetrate into the nuclei by these open poles. (2) Each nucleus moves to the central portion of the parasite, and one of them is located in the dorsal region and another in the ventral region and (3) the spindle is observed in the telophase [34]. Moreover, the parasite does not synchronize the nuclei division, and thus it is possible to find cells with three or four nuclei [35]. During the encystation process, the parasite mitosis still occurs; this is similar to what happens in the trophozoite vegetative form [36]. The nuclear division starts in the initial stages of encystation process through a semi-open mitosis. Bridges that originate by the nuclear membrane fusion connect the parental daughter nuclei. This interconnection between the nuclei remains intact while the parasite is in the cyst form; this is a characteristic of this stage in the *Giardia* life cycle [36].

Encysting cells show intranuclear inclusions that are morphologically similar to the ESVs and the ER membranes (**Figure 5c** and **d**), which may be a result of nuclear envelope folding. The presence of these inclusions could indicate intense ER activity since it forms from the outer nuclear membrane [33].

6. Encystment

The encystment (or encystation) is the given name for the parasite differentiation process of a trophozoite into a cyst (**Figure 6**). This process consists of several events and occurs in response to environmental or chemical stimuli. The chemical stimulus is a set of an alkaline pH, an increase of bile concentration and the presence of lactic acid released by bacteria that live in the gut [37]. The encystation process is a key for the parasite virulence mechanism and is responsible for the change to a resistant form that can survive in the outside environment for subsequent infection of a new host. This process also promotes the parasite immune evasion and is target to vaccine and drugs development [38, 39].

The encystation process is characterized by a gradual transformation of a flagellated trophozoite—which looks like a cut half pear—into a different structure called the cyst (**Figure 6**). The trophozoites lose their abilities to adhere, and there is a folding of the ventral disc, followed by its fragmentation [40]. The cell becomes rounded, internalizes the flagella as in an endocytic process and finally a filamentous layer involving the parasite creating the cyst wall (CW). Its superficial filaments connect cyst clusters [40]. Two layers form the CW: a filamentous layer and a membranous layer [41]. Biochemical analyses have focused on the filamentous layer, which is composed by 57% of proteins and 43% of carbohydrates [42].

The main protein components are the cyst wall proteins 1, 2 and 3 (CWPs 1, 2 and 3) and the HCNCp that belongs to a new class of *Giardia*'s proteins, known as cysteine-rich protein, differs from the variant surface proteins (VSP) [29]. The β-1,3-N-acetyl-D-galactosamine polymer (GalNAc) makes up almost 86% of the carbohydrates that compose the filaments layer of CW [42]. The GalNAc polymer forms the CW fibrils that are covered by protein clusters, such as the CWPs [43].

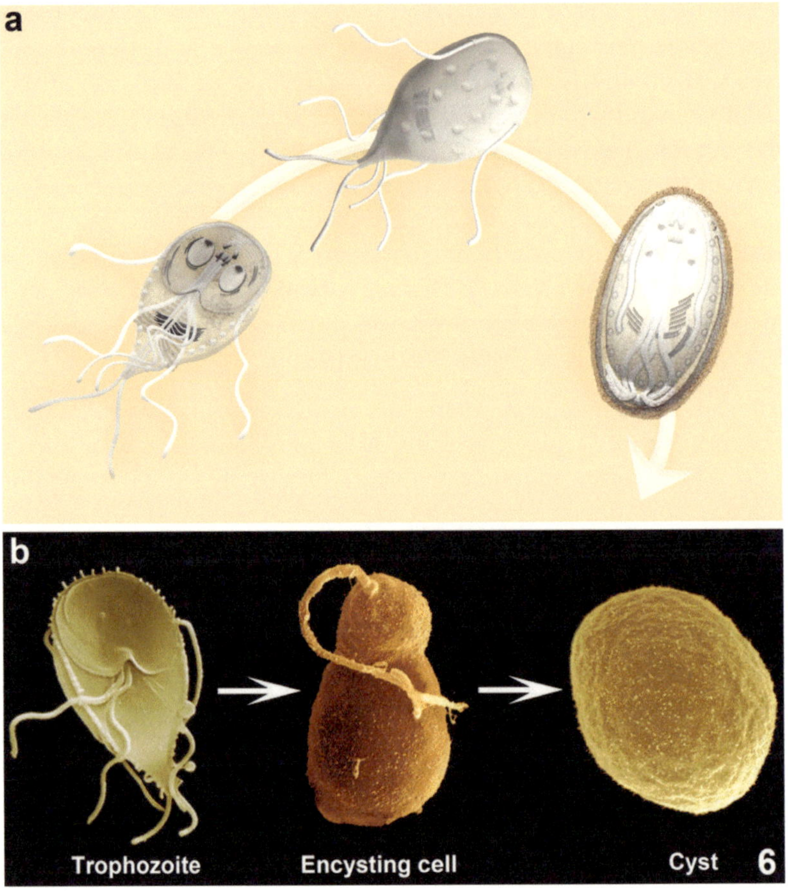

Figure 6. Encystation process of *G. intestinalis*. (a) Scheme of changes from trophozoite to a rounded oval cyst. (b) Scanning electron microscopy of encystation process showing the cell differentiation: the trophozoite internalizes the flagella, becoming oval. During encystation, the caudal flagella form a tail. At the end, the mature cyst presents a cyst wall and flagella are not seen anymore (unpublished).

6.1. Encystation vesicles

6.1.1. Encystation-specific vesicles (ESVs)

Before the formation of CW, in the beginning of the encystation process, large 1-μm vesicles known as encystation specific vesicles (ESVs) appear (**Figures 2c**, **5d**, **7–10**) [44]. The protein content of the ESVs is basically CWPs 1–3 (**Figures 7a** and **b**, **10**) that originate in the endoplasmic reticulum; afterwards, the encystation vesicles emerge from endoplasmic reticulum points (**Figures 7c** and **9a**) [45]. This mechanism is not fully understood; however, the available data points to two hypotheses: (1) the CW material concentrates in a specialized endoplasmic reticulum sub-compartment, and afterwards, a lateral segregation occurs [46] and/or (2) the CWPs transport to the ESVs through vesicles containing COPII followed by a homotypic fusion [47].

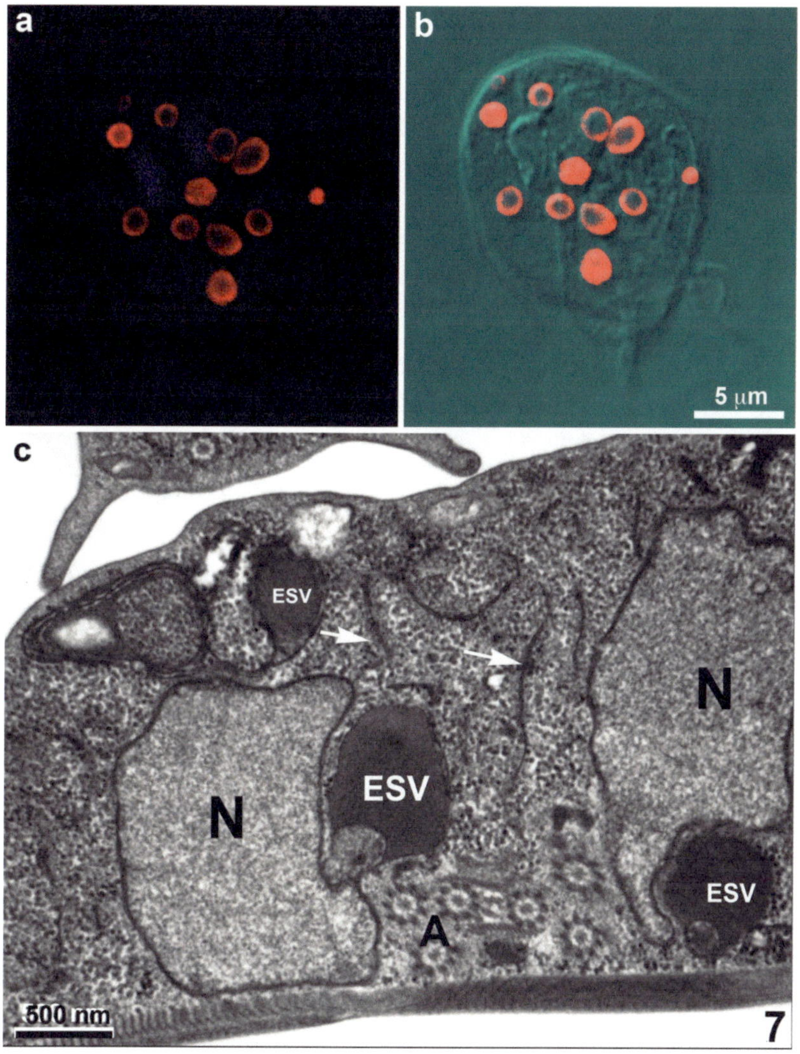

Figure 7. Encystation-specific vesicles (ESVs) during differentiation of *G. intestinalis* by confocal microscopy (a and b) and transmission electron microscopy (TEM) (c). (a and b) Immunofluorescence of the parasite induced to encyst *in vitro* for 21 h and labeled with an anti-CWP1 antibody against the cyst wall. In (c) ESVs are electron-dense, membrane-bounded vesicles. Note that some ESVs are close to the nuclei and endoplasmic reticulum (arrows). N, nuclei; A, axonemes (unpublished).

The ESVs maturation is less controversial: about 15–24 h post-encystment induction, before the CWP secretion, the ESVs recruit sequentially membrane peripheral proteins [48]. Thus, the ESVs and their content enter in a maturation way in which the CWPs are post-translationally modified. The presence of the protein disulfide isomerase 2 (PDI2) in ESVs indicates a post-translational mechanism [49] as well the CWP2 C terminal region cleavage by a specific encystation protease [50] and by the phosphorylation of newly synthesized CWPs [51].

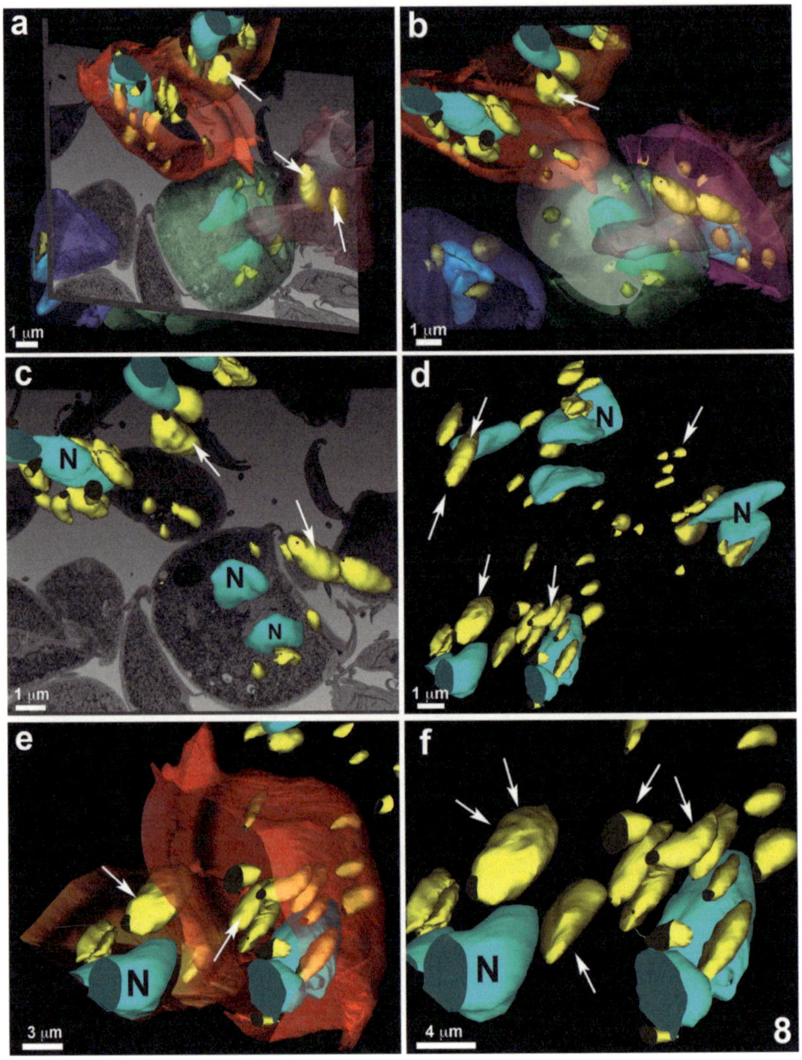

Figure 8. Three-dimensional reconstruction of encysting *G. intestinalis*. (a–f) Dual-beam microscopy and 3D reconstruction of 21-h encysted parasites. Seven parasites were reconstructed; ESVs are yellow (arrows) (Figs. a-b) and are distributed nearby the nuclei colored by light blue (N) (Figs. e–f). Cell membranes are in different colors (big contours) (unpublished).

6.1.2. Encystation carbohydrate-positive vesicles (ECVs)

For a long time, the understanding of how glycopolymers are transported to build the sugar portion of the CW remained an open question. This was mainly due to the lack of a marker that could track the carbohydrate portion of *Giardia*'s CW with strong specificity [52]. Some researchers used the *Dolichos biflorus* agglutinin (DBA) lectin, which has specificity to the GalNAc glycopolymer, to label the cyst wall of other parasites such as *Toxoplasma gondii* [53, 54]. Midlej and collaborators [55] used the DBA lectin as a tool to track the sugar moieties of *G. intestinalis* CW and were able to identify the encystation carbohydrate-positive vesicles

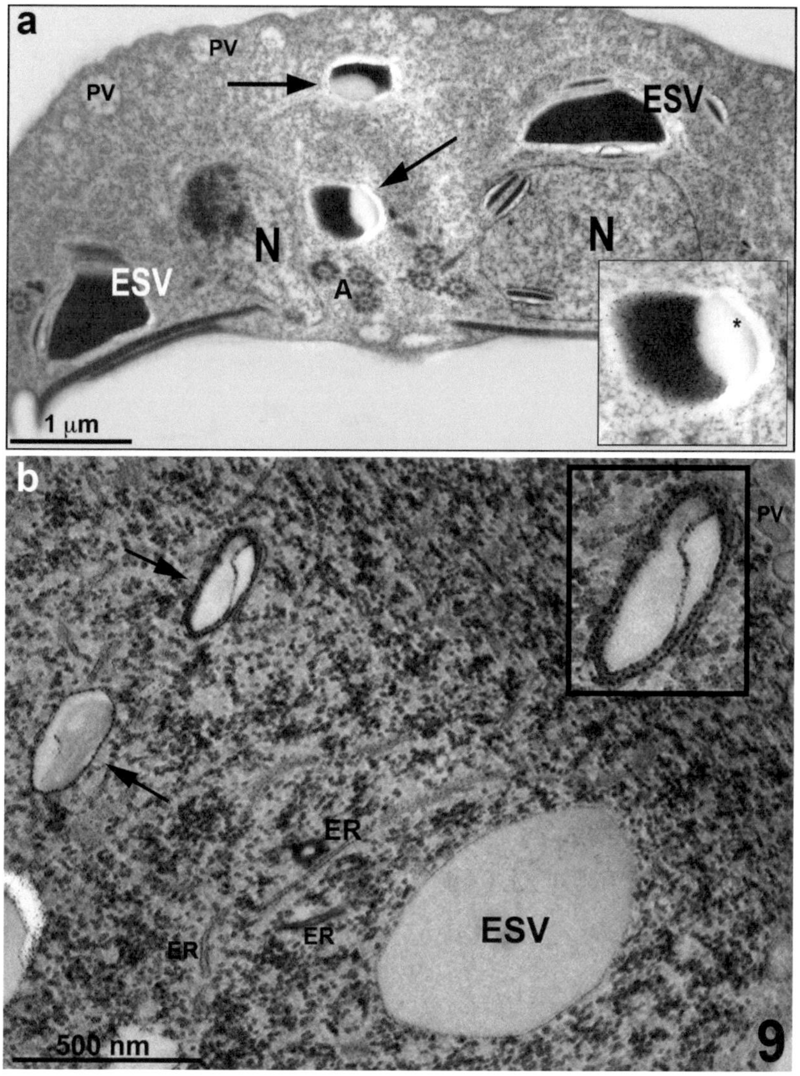

Figure 9. TEM images of *G. intestinalis* in process of encystation. (a) Immunolabeling with CWP1 antibody. Note the presence of two types of vesicles: electron dense (ESVs) and electron lucent (ECVs) (arrows). The ESVs (inset), which are juxtaposed to the ECVs (asterisks), present an intense labeling with anti-CWP1, whereas the ECVs present no labeling. (b) Cytochemistry for carbohydrates in encysted parasites: cell membranes, glycogen granules, the peripheral lumen and contents of the ECVs show a positive reaction (arrows), whereas the ESVs are negative (from Midlej et al. [55]).

(ECVs) (**Figures 9** and **10**). The ECVs are 0.2–2 μm membrane-bounded organelles (**Figure 9**). By electron microscopy, they are electron-lucent, whereas ESVs are electron dense (**Figure 9**). Moreover, the ECVs do not react with antibodies against CWPs (**Figure 10**) [55]. These vesicles are only in those encysting cells and are involved in the *Giardia's* CW biogenesis. The origin of ECVs seems to be related to the rough endoplasmic reticulum, because a budding vesicle was detected from this organelle in a similar way to what happens with the ESVs [56]. Thus, both

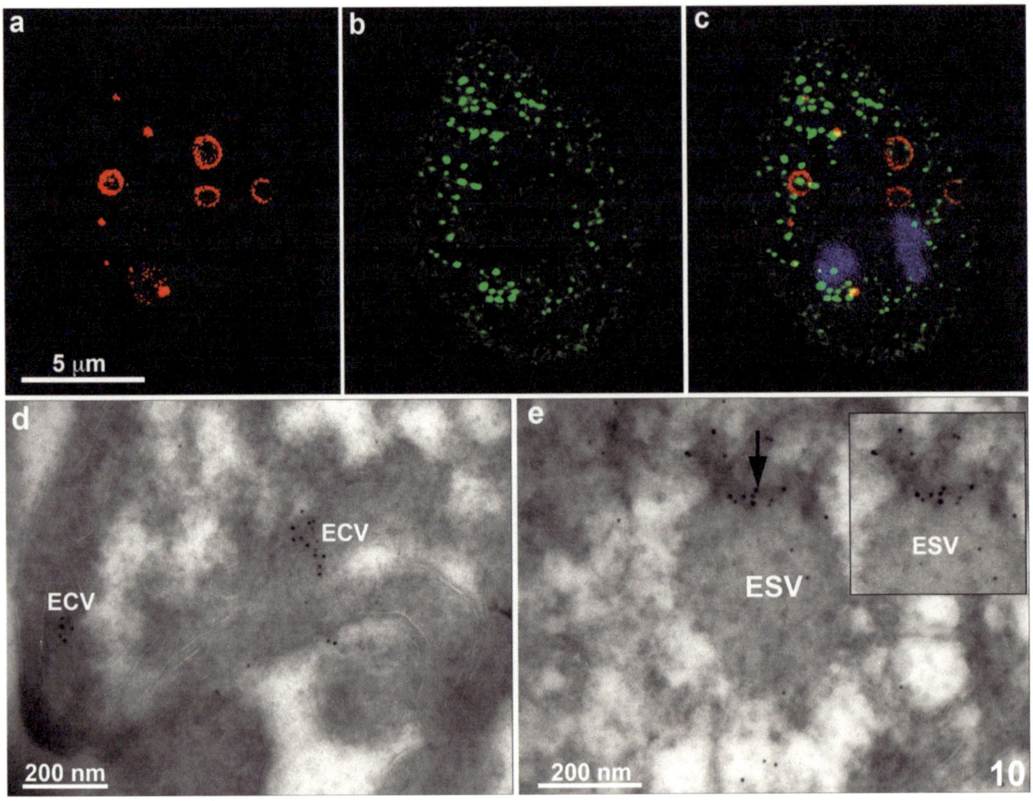

Figure 10. Immunolocalization of ECVs in encysting *Giardia*. DBA lectin was used to track the ECVs by immunofluorescence with confocal microscopy (a–c) and by cryo-immunogold in TEM microscopy (d and e). The ESVs were labeled with an anti-CWP1 antibody (a, c, d). The ESVs are red (a), while the ECVs are green (b). Note that the ECVs do not co-localized with the ESVs (c). The nuclei are blue. (d and e) Cryo-immunogold labeling with an anti-CWP1 antibody (gold with 5 nm) and the DBA lectin (gold with 10 nm). ECVs show a specific labeling for DBA (arrow)(Figs. c-e), whereas the ESVs (e) are with the anti-CWP1 antibody, with no labeling for the DBA lectin (inset). In the inset of figure e, an intense labeling for DBA is seen in ECV juxtaposed to the ESV (from Midlej et al. [55]).

secretion products are synthesized in the endoplasmic reticulum, budded together and are later separated and transported to the protozoan periphery to be secreted via exocytosis [55].

7. Mitosomes

Mitosomes are organelles described by Tovar and collaborators [57]. This name means "crypton" and was used to indicate it as reduced mitochondria. It is part of the mitochondria-related organelles as the hydrogenosomes found in *Trichomonas* [58]. Although the mitosomes are related to mitochondria, it lacks several mitochondrial characteristics and functions, such as ATP synthesis, the citric acid cycle, oxidative phosphorylation, heme biosynthesis, presence of DNA, lipid metabolism and the amino acid and urea cycles [59]. On the other hand, mitosomes present mitochondrial characteristics, such as biosynthesis of Fe-S clusters, presence of a TOM and TIM protein family transport machinery and a double membrane (**Figure 11a–c**) [60].

The mitosomes are small organelles, 200 nm in size, distributed over the cytoplasm, although some of them are placed between the flagellar axonemes. Because of that, they are divided into two distinct groups: the peripheral and central mitosomes (**Figure 11d** and **e**), which are dispersed in the cell and between nuclei, respectively [57]. The presence of an iron-sulfur complex (IscS and IscU proteins) makes its identification and characterization easier [61]. Mitosomes are also present, besides the IscS and IscU proteins, chaperones, such as Cnp60 and HSP70 [62]. During the encystation process, the mitosomes change their behavior, modulating Cpn60 and HSP70, and also alter their shape (**Figure 11d** and **e**) [62].

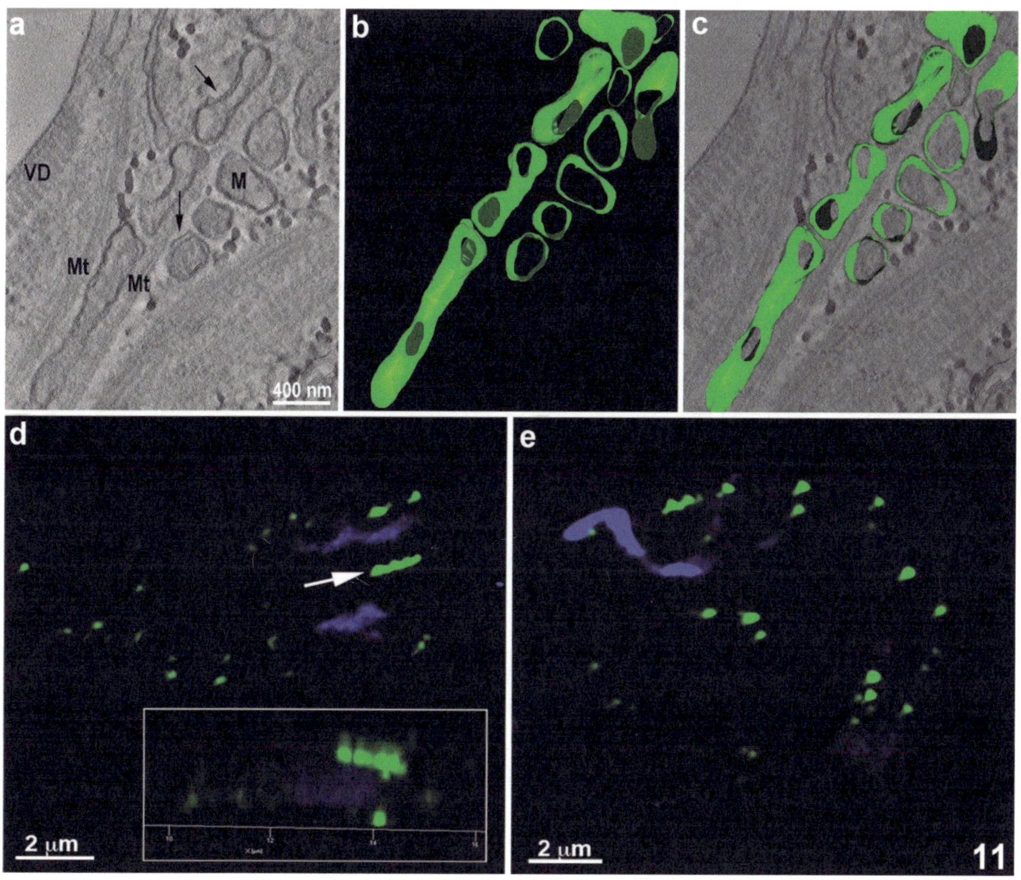

Figure 11. Mitosomes of *G. intestinalis*. Electron tomography (figures a–c) and super-resolution-structured illumination microscopy (SR-SIM) (figures d and e) of peripheral and central mitosomes. (a–c) Mitosomes in a non-encysted parasite are identified by their double-bound membrane (black arrows). Some mitosomes are elongated or ovoid organelles. (b) Three-dimensional reconstruction of mitosomes in green. (c) After reconstruction, the 3D model was placed on electron tomography micrograph. VD, ventral disc; M, mitosome; Mt., microtubules. (d and e) SR-SIM, vegetative cell (d) and cyst (e). Mitosomes are labeled using an antibody anti-IscU (green fluorescence). The super-resolution microscopy revealed that the central mitosome (white arrow) is seen as a unique tiny organelle between the nuclei (d). The spots of the central mitosome are better visualized in the inset, presenting a different axis angle (d). (e) Cyst mitosomes observed by SR-SIM. Nuclei are labeled with DAPI (blue) (from Midlej et al. [62]).

Thus, the current knowledge concerning mitosomes is still limited. There are a number of unanswered questions related to the biology of this organelle and its proteins as well as related to the importance of mitosomes in the parasite life cycle.

8. Golgi complex

There is still controversy regarding the presence of a Golgi complex in *G. intestinalis*. This organelle is usually characterized by the presence of several stacked cisternae, which are often located around the nucleus and close to the endoplasmic reticulum. Until now, an organelle that fits with these criteria has not been identified in *G. intestinalis*.

Some groups proposed a similarity between the ESVs and the Golgi complex [47, 52, 63–65] supported by: (1) COPI and COPII association with the ESVs [47]; (2) the ESVs are sensitive for Brefeldin A, a drug known to inhibits the anterograde Golgi cisternae movement [63]; (3) the ESVs dependence of GTPases Sar1 and Arf1 for biogenesis and maturation, respectively [64]. However, the ESVs present some characteristics that do not fit with those presented by a classical Golgi: (1) the ESVs appear only during the encystation process; (2) no classical Golgi markers such as GM130, galactosyl transferases or the trans-Golgi network marker Rab6 are present in the parasite; (3) the ESVs do not present morphological characteristics that define this organelle as a Golgi, in accordance with parameters that have been well defined for many years. This is considered a strong argument for the absence of a typical Golgi in *G. intestinalis* [65]. Thus, it is hard to directly test if the ESVs are in fact similar to the Golgi complex or if this organelle evolved independently.

9. Final remarks

The endomembrane system of *Giardia* is well adapted to changes that are encountered in the gut environment and outside the warm and nutritious body. The cysts ensure the efficacy of the parasite in host colonization. Despite the low complexity of organelles and machinery involved, *G. intestinalis* constitutes a model for the investigation of synthesis, transport and assembly of simple but highly effective biopolymers [43, 52].

There are several questions to be answered regarding the biology of Giardia—for example, the right pathway of endocytic and exocytic materials, the formation of the cyst wall, each protein segregation and polymerization in the formation of the cyst wall, the glycosylation phenomena of secreted proteins, the role of each nucleus in the whole process of the Giardia life cycle, among others.

Acknowledgements

This work was supported by the Conselho Nacional de Desenvolvimento Científico e Tecnológico (CNPq), Financiadora de Estudos e Projetos (FINEP), Fundação Carlos Chagas Filho de Amparo a Pesquisa do Estado do Rio de Janeiro (FAPERJ), Coordenação de Aperfeiçoamento de Pessoal de Nível Superior (CAPES) and Programa de Núcleos de Excelência (PRONEX).

Author details

Victor Midlej[1,3,4]*, Wanderley de Souza[1,3,4] and Marlene Benchimol[1,2,3,4]

*Address all correspondence to: marlenebenchimol@gmail.com or vmidlej@hotmail.com

1 Instituto de Biofísica Carlos Chagas Filho, Universidade Federal do Rio de Janeiro, Brazil

2 Universidade UNIGRANRIO, Rua Prof. José de Souza Herdy, Brazil

3 Instituto Nacional de Ciência e Tecnologia em Biologia Estrutural e Bioimagens-INBEB, Rio de Janeiro, Brazil

4 Centro Nacional de Bioimagens-CENABIO, Rio de Janeiro, Brazil

References

[1] Blanchard R. Remarques sur le megastome intestinal. Bulletin de la Société Zoologique de France. 1888;**13**:18

[2] Dobell C. The discovery of the intestinal protozoa of man. Proceedings of the Royal Society of Medicine. 1920;**13**:1-15

[3] Lambl W. Mikroskopische untersuchungen der Darmexcrete. Vierteljahrsschr Prakst Heikunde. 1859;**61**:1-58

[4] Adam RD. The biology of *Giardia* spp. Microbiological Reviews. 1991;**55**:706-732

[5] Karanis P, Kourenti C, Smith H. Waterborne transmission of protozoan parasites: a worldwide review of outbreaks and lessons learnt. Journal of Water and Health. 2007;**5**: 1-38. DOI: 10.1016/j.watres.2011.10.013

[6] Ludwig KM, Frei F, Alvares Filho F, Ribeiro-Paes JT. Correlation between sanitation conditions and intestinal parasitosis in the population of Assis, State of São Paulo. Revista da Sociedade Brasileira de Medicina Tropical. 1999;**2**:547-555. DOI: 10.1590/S0037-86821999000500013

[7] Escobedo AA, Almirall P, Robertson LJ, Franco RM, Hanevik K. Giardiasis: the ever-present threat of a neglected disease. Infectious Disorders Drug Targets. 2010;**10**:329-348. DOI: 10.2174/187152610793180821

[8] Kramer MH, Herwaldt BL, Craun GF, Calderon RL, Juranek DD. Surveillance for waterborne disease outbreaks—United States, 1993–1994. MMWR. CDC Surveillance Summaries. 1996;**45**:1-33. DOI: 10.1016/j.watres.2011.10.013

[9] Samuelson J. Why metronidazole is active against both bacteria and parasites. Antimicrobial Agents and Chemotherapy. 1999;**43**:1533-1541

[10] Cavalier-Smith T. The neomuran revolution and phagotrophic origin of eukaryotes and cilia in the light of intracellular coevolution and a revised tree of life. Cold Spring Harbor Perspectives in Biology. 2014;**6**:a016006. DOI: 10.1101/cshperspect.a016006

[11] Mast FD, Barlow LD, Rachubinski RA, Dacks JB. Evolutionary mechanisms for establishing eukaryotic cellular complexity. Trends in Cell Biology. 2014;**24**:435-442. DOI: 10.1016/j.tcb.2014.02.003

[12] Lloyd D, Harris JC, Maroulis S, Wadley R, Ralphs JR, Hann AC, Turner MP, Edwards MR. The "primitive" microaerophile *Giardia intestinalis* (syn. lamblia, duodenalis) has specialized membranes with electron transport and membrane-potential-generating functions. Microbiologica. 2002;**148**:1349-1354. DOI: 10.1099/00221287-148-5-1349

[13] Wampfler PB, Tosevski V, Nanni P, Spycher C, Hehl AB. Proteomics of secretory and endocytic organelles in *Giardia lamblia*. PLoS One. 2014;**9**:e94089. DOI: 10.1371/journal.pone.0094089

[14] Feely DE, Dyer JK. Localization of acid phosphatase activity in *Giardia lamblia* and *Giardia muris* trophozoites. The Journal of Protozoology. 1987;**34**:80-83

[15] Kattenbach WM, Pimenta PFP, De Souza W, Pinto Da Silva P. *Giardia duodenalis*: A freeze-fracture, fracture- flip and cytochemistry study. Parasitology Research. 1991;**77**:651-658. DOI: 10.1007/BF00928678

[16] Meyer EA. Giardia as an organism. In: Thompson RCA, editor. Giardia: From Molecules to Disease. 1st ed. Oxford: CAB International; 1994. p. 3-13

[17] Lanfredi-Rangel A, Attias M, De Carvalho TM, Kattenbach WM, De Souza W. The peripheral vesicles of trophozoites of the primitive protozoan *Giardia lamblia* may correspond to early and late endosomes and to lysosomes. Journal of Structural Biology. 1998;**123**:225-235. DOI: 10.1006/jsbi.1998.4035

[18] Tai JH, Ong SJ, Chang SC, Su HM. Giardiavirus enters *Giardia lamblia* WB trophozoite via endocytosis. Experimental Parasitology. 1993;**76**:165-174. DOI: 10.1006/expr.1993.1019

[19] Abodeely M, Dubois KN, Hehl A, Stefanic S, Sajid M, De Souza W, Attias M, Engel JC, Hsieh I, Fetter RD, Mckerrow JH. A contiguous compartment functions as endoplasmic reticulum and endosome/lysosome in *Giardia lamblia*. Eukaryotic Cell. 2009;**8**:1665-1676. DOI: 10.1128/EC.00123-09

[20] Gaechter V, Schraner E, Wild P, Hehl AB. The single dynamin family protein in the primitive protozoan *Giardia lamblia* is essential for stage conversion and endocytic transport. Traffic. 2008;**9**:57-71. DOI: 10.1111/j.1600-0854.2007.00657.x

[21] Rivero MR, Vranych CV, Bisbal M, Maletto BA, Ropolo AS, Touz MC. Adaptor protein 2 regulates receptor-mediated endocytosis and cyst formation in *Giardia lamblia*. The Biochemical Journal. 2010;**428**:33-45. DOI: 10.1042/BJ20100096

[22] Zumthor JP, Cernikova L, Rout S, Kaech A, Faso C, Hehl AB. Static clathrin assemblies at the peripheral vacuole-plasma membrane interface of the parasitic protozoan *Giardia lamblia*. PLoS Pathogens. 2016;**12**:e1005756. DOI: 10.1371/journal.ppat.1005756

[23] Soltys BJ, Falah M, Gupta RS. Identification of endoplasmic reticulum in the primitive eukaryote *Giardia lamblia* using cryoelectron microscopy and antibody to Bip. Journal of Cell Science. 1996;**109**:1909-1917

[24] Knodler LA, Noiva R, Mehta K, Mccaffery JM, Aley SB, Svärd SG, Nystul TG, Reiner DS, Silberman JD, Gillin FD. Novel protein-disulfide isomerases from the early-diverging protist *Giardia lamblia*. The Journal of Biological Chemistry. 1999;**274**:29805-29811. DOI: 10.1074/jbc.274.42.29805

[25] Banerjee S, Vishwanath P, Cui J, Kelleher DJ, Gilmore R, Robbins PW, Samuelson J. The evolution of N-glycan-dependent endoplasmic reticulum quality control factors for glycoprotein folding and degradation. Proceedings of the National Academy of Sciences of the United States of America. 2007;**104**:11676-11681. DOI: 10.1073/pnas.0704862104

[26] Banerjee S, Cui J, Robbins PW, Samuelson J. Use of Giardia, which appears to have a single nucleotide-sugar transporter for UDP-GlcNAc, to identify the UDP-Glc transporter of entamoeba. Molecular and Biochemical Parasitology. 2008;**159**:44-53. DOI: 10.1016/j.molbiopara.2008.01.004

[27] Svard SG, Rafferty C, McCaffery JM, Smith MW, Reiner DS, Gillin FD. A signal recognition particle receptor gene from the early-diverging eukaryote, *Giardia lamblia*. Molecular and Biochemical Parasitology. 1999;**98**:253-264

[28] Morrison HG, McArthur AG, Gillin FD, Aley SB, Adam RD, Olsen GJ, Best AA, Cande WZ, Chen F, Cipriano MJ, Davids BJ, Dawson SC, Elmendorf HG, Hehl AB, Holder ME, Huse SM, Kim UU, Lasek-Nesselquist E, Manning G, Nigam A, Nixon JE, Palm D, Passamaneck NE, Prabhu A, Reich CI, Reiner DS, Samuelson J, Svard SG, Sogin ML. Genomic minimalism in the early diverging intestinal parasite *Giardia lamblia*. Science. 2007;**317**:1921-1926. DOI: 10.1126/science.1143837

[29] Davids BJ, Reiner DS, Birkeland SR, Preheim SP, Cipriano MJ, McArthur AG, Gillin FD. A new family of giardial cysteine-rich non-VSP protein genes and a novel cyst protein. PLoS One. 2006;**1**:e44. DOI: 10.1371/journal.pone.0000044

[30] Shen HE, Cao L, Li J, Tian XF, Yang ZH, Wang Y, Tian YN, Lu SQ. Visualization of chromosomes in the binucleate intestinal parasite *Giardia lamblia*. Parasitology Research. 2011;**109**:1439-1445. DOI: 10.1007/s00436-011-2392-6

[31] Alberts B, Johnson A, Lewis J, Raff M, Roberts K, Walther P. Molecular Biology of The Cell. 4th. New York: Garland Science; 2002; 712 p. DOI: 10.1002/bmb.2003.494031049999

[32] Benchimol M. A new set of vesicles in *Giardia lamblia*. Experimental Parasitology. 2002;**102**:30-37. DOI: 10.1016/S0014-4894(02)00142-X

[33] Benchimol M. Participation of the adhesive disc during karyokinesis in *Giardia lamblia*. Biology of the Cell. 2004;**96**:291-301. DOI: 10.1016/j.biolcel.2004.01.007

[34] Sagolla MS, Dawson SC, Mancuso JJ, Cande WZ. Three dimensional analysis of mitosis and cytokinesis in the binucleate parasite *Giardia intestinalis*. Journal of Cell Science. 2006;**119**:4889-4900. DOI: 10.1242/jcs.03276

[35] Benchimol M. Mitosis in *Giardia lamblia*: multiple modes of cytokinesis. Protist. 2004;**155**: 33-44. DOI: 10.1078/1434461000162

[36] Jiráková K, Kulda J, Nohýnková E. How nuclei of Giardia pass through cell differentiation: Semi-open mitosis followed by nuclear interconnection. Protist. 2012;**163**:465-479. DOI: 10.1016/j.protis.2011.11.008

[37] Gillin FD, Boucher SE, Rossi SS, Reiner DS. *Giardia lamblia*: The roles of bile, lactic acid, and pH in the completion of the life cycle in vitro. Experimental Parasitology. 1989;**69**:164-174. DOI: 10.1016/0014-4894(89)90185-9

[38] Lee P, Faubert GM. Oral immunization of BALB/c mice by intragastric delivery of *Streptococcus gordonii* expressing Giardia cyst wall protein 2 decreases cyst shedding in challenged mice. FEMS Microbiology Letters. 2006;**265**:225-236. DOI: 10.1111/j.1574-6968.2006.00490.x

[39] Lee P, Faubert GM. Expression of the *Giardia lamblia* cyst wall protein 2 in *Lactococcus lacti*s. Microbiology. 2006;**152**:1981-1990. DOI: 10.1099/mic.0.28877-0

[40] Midlej V, Benchimol M. *Giardia lamblia* behavior during encystment: How morphological changes in shape occur. Parasitology International. 2009;**58**:72-80. DOI: 10.1016/j.parint.2008.11.002

[41] Erlandsen SL, Bemrick WJ, Pawley J. High resolution electron microscopic evidence for the filamentous structure of the cyst wall in *Giardia muris* and *Giardia duodenalis*. The Journal of Parasitology. 1989;**75**:787-797

[42] Gerwig GJ, Van Kuik JA, Leeflang BR, Kamerling JP, Vliegenthart JF, Karr CD, Jarroll EL. The Giardia intestinalis filamentous cyst wall contains a novel beta(s1-3)-N-acetyl-D-galactosamine polymer: A structural and conformational study. Glycobiology. 2002;**12**:499-505. DOI: 10.1093/glycob/cwf059

[43] Chatterjee A, Carpentieri A, Ratner DM, Bullitt E, Costello CE, Robbins PW, Samuelson J. Giardia cyst wall protein 1 is a lectin that binds curled fibrils of the GalNAc homopolymer. PLoS Pathogens. 2010;**6**:e1001059. DOI: 10.1371/journal.ppat.1001059

[44] Faubert G, Reiner DS, Gillin FD. *Giardia lamblia*: Regulation of secretory vesicle formation and loss of ability to reattach during encystation in vitro. Experimental Parasitology. 1991;**72**:345-354

[45] Hehl AB, Marti M. Secretory protein trafficking in *Giardia intestinalis*. Molecular Microbiology. 2004;**53**:19-28. DOI: 10.1111/j.1365-2958.2004.04115.x

[46] Lanfredi-Rangel A, Attias M, Reiner DS, Gillin FD, De Souza W. Fine structure of the biogenesis of *Giardia lamblia* encystation secretory vesicles. Journal of Structural Biology. 2003;**143**:153-163. DOI: 10.1016/S1047-8477(03)00123-0

[47] Marti M, Li Y, Schraner EM, Wild P, Kohler P, Hehl AB. The secretory apparatus of an ancient eukaryote: Protein sorting to separate export pathways occurs before formation of transient Golgi-like compartments. Molecular Biology of the Cell. 2003;**14**:1433-1447. DOI: 10.1091/mbc.E02-08-0467

[48] Marti M, Regos A, Li Y, Em S, Wild P, Muller N, Lg K, Ab H. An ancestral secretory apparatus in the protozoan parasite *Giardia intestinalis*. The Journal of Biological Chemistry. 2003;**278**:24837-24848. DOI: 10.1091/mbc.E02-08-0467

[49] Davids BJ, Mehta K, Fesus L, McCaffery JM, Gillin FD. Dependence of *Giardia lamblia* encystation on novel transglutaminase activity. Molecular and Biochemical Parasitology. 2004;**136**:173-180. DOI: 10.1016/j.molbiopara.2004.03.011

[50] Touz MC, Nores MJ, Slavin I, Carmona C, Conrad JT, Mowatt MR, Nash TE, Coronel CE, Lujan HD. The activity of a developmentally regulated cysteine proteinase is required for cyst wall formation in the primitive eukaryote *Giardia lamblia*. The Journal of Biological Chemistry. 2002;**277**:8474-8481. DOI: 10.1074/jbc.M110250200

[51] Slavin I, Saura A, Carranza PG, Touz MC, Nores MJ, Lujan HD. Dephosphorylation of cyst wall proteins by a secreted lysosomal acid phosphatase is essential for excystation of *Giardia lamblia*. Molecular and Biochemical Parasitology. 2002;**122**:95-98. DOI: 10.1016/S0166-6851(02)00065-8

[52] Konrad C, Spycher C, Hehl AB. Selective condensation drives partitioning and sequential secretion of cyst wall proteins in differentiating *Giardia lamblia*. PLoS Pathogens. 2010;**6**: e1000835. DOI: 10.1371/journal.ppat.1000835

[53] Zhang YW, Halonen SK, Ma YF, Tanowtiz HB, Weiss LM. A purification method for enrichment of the *Toxoplasma gondii* cyst wall. Journal of Neuroparasitology. 2010; pii: N101001. DOI: 10.4303/jnp/N101001

[54] Tobin C, Pollard A, Knoll L. *Toxoplasma gondii* cyst wall formation in activated bone marrow-derived macrophages and bradyzoite conditions. Journal of Visualized Experiments. 2010; pii:2091. DOI: 10.3791/2091

[55] Midlej V, Meinig I, de Souza W, Benchimol M. A new set of carbohydrate-positive vesicles in encysting *Giardia lamblia*. Protist 2013;**164**:261–271. DOI: 10.1016/j.protis.2012.11.001

[56] Reiner DS, McCaffery M, Gillin FD. Sorting of cyst wall proteins to a regulated secretory pathway during differentiation of the primitive eukaryote, *Giardia lamblia*. European Journal of Cell Biology. 1990;**53**:142-153

[57] Tovar J, León-Avila G, Sánchez LB, Sutak R, Tachezy J, van der Giezen M, Hernández M, Müller M, Lucocq JM. Mitochondrial remnant organelles of Giardia function in iron-sulphur protein maturation. Nature 2003;**426**:172–176. DOI: 10.1038/nature01945

[58] Tovar J, Fischer A, Clark CG. The mitosome, a novel organelle related to mitochondria in the amitochondrial parasite *Entamoeba histolytica*. Molecular Microbiology. 1999;**32**:1013-1021. DOI: 10.1046/j.1365-2958.1999.01414.x

[59] Makiuchi T, Nozaki T. Highly divergent mitochondrion-related organelles in anaerobic parasitic protozoa. Biochimie. 2014;**100**:3-17. DOI: 10.1016/j.biochi.2013.11.018

[60] Tachezy J, Smid O. Mitosomes in parasitic protists. In: Tachezy J, editor. Hydrogenosomes and Mitosomes: Mitochondria of Anaerobic Eukaryotes. 1st ed. Berlin: Springer-Verlag; 2008. p. 201-230

[61] Tachezy J, Sanchez LB, Muller M. Mitochondrial type iron-sulfur cluster 15 assembly in the amitochondriate eukaryotes *Trichomonas vaginalis* and *Giardia intestinalis*, as indicated by the phylogeny of IscS. Molecular Biology and Evolution. 2001;**18**:1919-1928

[62] Midlej V, Penha L, Silva R, de Souza W, Benchimol M. Mitosomal chaperone modulation during the life cycle of the pathogenic protist *Giardia intestinalis*. European Journal of Cell Biology 2016;**95**:531–542. DOI: 10.1016/j.ejcb.2016.08.005

[63] Luján HD, Marotta A, Mowatt MR, Sciaky N, Lippincottschwartz J, Nash TE. Developmental induction of Golgi structure and function in the primitive eukaryote *Giardia lamblia*. The Journal of Biological Chemistry. 1995;**270**:4612-4618. DOI: 10.1074/jbc.270.9.4612

[64] Stefanic S, Morf L, Kulangara C, Regös A, Sonda S, Schraner E, Spycher C, Wild P, Hehl AB. Neogenesis and maturation of transient Golgi-like cisternae in a simple eukaryote. Journal of Cell Science. 2009;**122**:2846-2856. DOI: 10.1242/jcs.049411

[65] Ebneter JA, Heusser SD, Schraner EM, Hehl AB, Faso C. Cyst wall-protein-1 is fundamental for Golgi-like organelle neogenesis and cyst wall biosynthesis in *Giardia lamblia*. Nature Communications. 2016;**15**:13859. DOI: 10.1038/ncomms13859

Chapter 7

Loop-Mediated Isothermal Amplification: An Advanced Method for the Detection of *Giardia*

Carmen Gallas-Lindemann, Poornima Sureshkumar,
Michael J. Noack and Isaia Sotiriadou

Additional information is available at the end of the chapter

http://dx.doi.org/10.5772/intechopen.70804

Abstract

This chapter provides a reliable and quick method for detection of *Giardia duodenalis* (which causes a dangerous diarrheal disease), prevention of further spreading, identification of the source of contamination, and eventually minimize health risk and economic damage normally caused by an outbreak. The loop-mediated isothermal amplification (LAMP) method is based on the enrichment of parasite-specific nucleotide sequences, similar to PCR, but it is significantly faster and less susceptible to interference. Here, we give an overview of how we developed this method, and using the example of *G. duodenalis* as a water-associated pathogen, we present an optimized examination scheme for its detection in water. For this purpose, we have analyzed data from extensive electronic libraries PubMed®/MEDLINE®, filtered out relevant articles with a keyword search, and summarized them. The number of publications on LAMP method has generally increased steadily since its first report in 2000. LAMP, used for detection of *Giardia*, especially surpasses all other methods due to the high specificity, sensitivity, robustness, and cost effectiveness. The ever-increasing number of publications on application of LAMP is similar to the development of PCR in the 1990s of the last century. Certainly, the method will be further developed in future, but it already offers many advantages over other methods for effective detection of *G. duodenalis* infections and will therefore certainly gain in popularity.

Keywords: loop mediated isothermal amplification, molecular detection, water, feces

1. Introduction

Among diarrheal diseases, Giardiasis induced by the protozoan parasite *Giardia duodenalis* plays a distinct role for a variety of reasons. Infections of humans and animals with the often overlooked protozoan parasite *Giardia duodenalis* have been reported worldwide. Giardiasis is mainly contracted with the consumption of food and drinking water contaminated with cysts—the environmentally resistant and dormant form of the parasite. *Giardia* cysts are excreted by livestock, wild, and companion animals. These cysts are equipped to survive in extreme and adverse conditions for a long time. The main route of infection is through spreading by water. Giardiasis often occurs as outbreaks, with devastating consequences on human health causing vast economic damage. And most importantly, prophylaxis in the form of drugs or vaccines is impossible. Unfortunately, the inability to involve improved, sensitive, and specific ways for rapid and reliable detection of *Giardia* using microscopic and molecular methods in different matrixes hamper the tracking of this parasite in the environment as well as in patients. For public health, frequent monitoring of water sources using LAMP as the preferred tool is quite effective in both accuracy and costs and can help to detect the parasite source at the earliest possible to avoid outbreaks.

1.1. *Giardia duodenalis:* genetic assemblages and hosts

Giardia is a Diplomonadida, flagellated protozoan with global distribution. The names *G. duodenalis, G. lamblia, and G. intestinalis* are the species names interchangeably used in current literature referring to the same organism. Based on genetic, structural, and biochemical data, they are systematically classified; *Giardia* belongs to phylum: Metamonada, subphylum: Trichozoa, superclass: Eopharyngia, class: Trepomonadea, subclass: Diplozoa, order: Giardiida, and family: Giardiidae [1, 2].

Anthony van Leeuwenhoek documented the genus in 1681 for the first time when he microscopically examined his own stool due to his continuous diarrheal sickness. In 1859, Lambl provided a detailed description of the trophozoite and the genus was named Lambl in honor of his work. Until 1879, the cyst stage of the life cycle was completely unknown awaiting Grassi to describe the robust parasitic stage that did not contain flagella (cysts) [3]. In order to give credit to the French zoologist Alfred Giard, Stiles changed the former name (genus and specific epithet) to *Giardia* [4] in 1915.

The *Giardia* genus can be divided into six different species: *G. duodenalis, G. agilis, G. muris, G. psittaci, G. ardae,* and *G. microti. G. duodenalis* can furthermore be divided into assemblages and subassemblages [5, 6]. Eight different *G. duodenalis* assemblages have been delineated (A–H) so far, of which assemblages A (subassemblages AI and AII) and B (subassemblages BIII and BIV) are mainly virulent for humans and are often referred to as "zoonotic" assemblages [6, 7]. Narrow host-adapted specificity has been found in assemblages C and D; dogs and canines with assemblage E and domestic livestock (cats) with assemblage F [5, 8]. Assemblage G is associated with rats and mice, whereas assemblage H infects gray seals and gulls [5].

1.2. The *Giardia* life cycle

The *Giardia* life cycle begins with the oral ingestion of a few cysts (ovoid, about 15 × 9 μm × 3 μm), which are resistant under environmental conditions retaining the infectious nature and are transmitted through contaminated water, food, or fecal-oral route (hands or fomites)

[9, 10]. Acknowledging the resilience of these cysts, the parasite is highly virulent; only 1–10 cysts are capable of causing giardiasis [11]. Following an oral ingestion, the low pH of the stomach acid induces excystation (rupture of the cysts) and duplication (asexual replication) of the cell into two binucleated trophozoites. The process of excystation involves the activation of flagella pushing itself out through the cyst wall induced by the proteolytic activity in the duodenum. Simultaneously, the trophozoite undergoes an asexual duplication resulting in every single cyst producing two trophozoites. The trophozoites attach themselves to the duodenal epithelium with their ventral sucking disk and remain within the lumen of the host's proximal small intestine where they are nutritioned by phagocytosis on the dorsal side of the trophozoite. Freely moving or being attached to the mucosa by a ventral sucking disk, they multiply asexually by longitudinal binary fission resulting in manifold reproduction leading to an invasive growth of the trophozoites in the intestine. Trophozoites at the rectum form a robust cyst wall. The trigger for this encystment is still unclear. The process seems to be a result of exposure to and induction by bile salts, fatty acids, and a more alkaline environment. The trophozoite retracts the flagella and division of the nuclei follows before the cysts are excreted with feces.

1.3. Symptoms of the disease

Giardia has a global distribution and is a major contributor to the enormous burden of diarrheal diseases [5, 12, 13]. Giardiasis is a self-limiting disease in immunocompetent individuals with an incubation period of a few days up to 3 weeks. The clinical manifestation is between 1 and 12 days, rarely exceeding 2 weeks [14–16]. Clinically, asymptomatic giardiasis in immunocompetent individual is possible and is frequently associated with excretion of cysts, which however cannot be avoided. Apart from the assemblage, the symptomatic course of infection is confined to be more susceptible in children and elderly/aged people due to their immune incompetence and other host factors [17]. The main symptoms are diarrhea, bloating, weight loss, malabsorption, flatulence, abdominal cramps, nausea, vomiting, fatigue, anorexia, and chills [18–20]. Treatment with drugs is possible within the course of the disease or in chronic conditions. However, preventive vaccination is unavailable [21, 22].

1.4. Transmission routes of giardiasis

The transmission of cysts is possible by the fecal-oral route, through contaminated food or via water-based transmission. *Giardia* cysts are excreted by livestock, wild, and companion animals and are equipped to survive in extreme and adverse conditions for a long time. The likelihood of distribution and consequently the transmission of *Giardia* cysts shed through feces of wild and/or domestic animals that are evident especially after heavy rainfall or river flooding. Such environmental factors favor their transfer to aquifers, local privately farmed gardens, and open-air greenhouses. Waterborne distribution is estimated to be the main source of infection according to various studies of recent years [12, 13, 23]. The food-borne transmission to humans as well as through consumption of packed salads and/or green leaves by infected food-handlers has been reported [24, 25]. Person-to-person contact among schoolchildren attending day care centers and crosscontamination from the staff to their households are also possible and have a significant epidemiological impact [26–28].

1.5. Epidemiology

The Robert Koch Institute (RKI) in Berlin is the only public health institute in Germany as well as a global health hub publishing weekly reports about illnesses in the German Epidemiological Bulletin. In 2009 and 2010, about 3500–4000 cases of giardiasis were reported [29]. In 2016, the reported *Giardia* cases were 522, whereas during the first 8 weeks of 2017, the reported cases were 415 equaling to about 50 giardiasis incidences per week [30]. In industrial countries, *G. duodenalis* often occurs after the holiday seasons through returning travelers from foreign countries. The post-travel, persistent diarrheal symptoms in patients are most likely related to giardiasis, which is why it is also called "traveler's disease" [31]. Especially, backpackers transmit the parasite to their homes after returning.

In sub-Saharan Africa (SSA), millions of people die of parasitic diseases annually. This includes neglected tropical diseases (NTDs). The geohelminths (soil-transmitted helminths [STHs]) and the intestinal *G. duodenalis* parasite alone infect hundreds of millions of people in SSA [32, 33].

According to the 2016 Statistical Yearbook of United Nation's High Commissioner for Refugees (UNHCR), forcibly displaced people exceeded the number of 65 million worldwide [34]. Until end of January 2016, more than 60,000 registered unaccompanied minor refugees (UMRs) were living in Germany, of which 1248 UMRs between January 2014 and December 2015 underwent an infectious disease screening. Interestingly, 29.2% (364 cases) were infected with more than one intestinal parasite and 7.6% of whom (95 cases) were diagnosed with *G. duodenalis* by immunofluorescence microscopy [35].

2. Database search and inclusion criteria

To ascertain the progress of the LAMP assay since it was developed by Natomi et al. [36] and further evolved by Negamine et al. [37], we conducted a database analysis by keyword search with a special focus on the genus *Giardia*. Two independent reviewers identified the records through PubMed®/MEDLINE®, the database which is considered to be the global literature, the most reliable source of literature search, and a relevant publication retrieval. Two reviewers independently extracted the data and independently assessed the methodological quality. To our best knowledge, this review aimed to assess all literature wherein the LAMP assay was developed and/or applied for detection of *Giardia* in the scientific field. The extraction of relevant literature and appraisal of the finally listed work was carried out up to March 2017. To collect precise information, the comprehensive search entailed the evaluation of published articles including full texts in the English language and those meeting the inclusion criteria were considered to be appropriate after a critical review. Our search showed one article published in the Turkish language also. We directly contacted the authors who transmitted the electronic text to us. We were able to assess the contents of the article with a translator's help. The terms "loop-mediated isothermal amplification," "loop-mediated isothermal amplification (and) *Giardia*," "LAMP," "LAMP (and) *Giardia*," "polymerase chain reaction," "polymerase chain reaction (and) *Giardia*," "PCR," and "PCR (and) *Giardia*" were entered into the search box, and the articles were processed for further data extraction.

2.1. Results of the literature search

In total, 1850 (0.36%) of extracted articles showed for the term "loop-mediated isothermal amplification" in comparison with 512,447 for "polymerase chain reaction." The LAMP assay was first published in 2000 with a continuous increase in the following years. Until now, LAMP assays have reached the highest level in 2015 with 271 articles published, and thus far until end of March 2017, 110 articles (extrapolated ~440) have been published, which explains the increasing tendency (**Diagram 1**).

Out of 13 LAMP-related articles dealing with the detection of *Giardia*, only six articles were found related to the source/medium: water. Most of the published papers are for the purpose of method evaluation or detection of the targets in patient samples like blood, tissue, and feces. LAMP in water samples was successfully applied for *Giardia* in five articles.

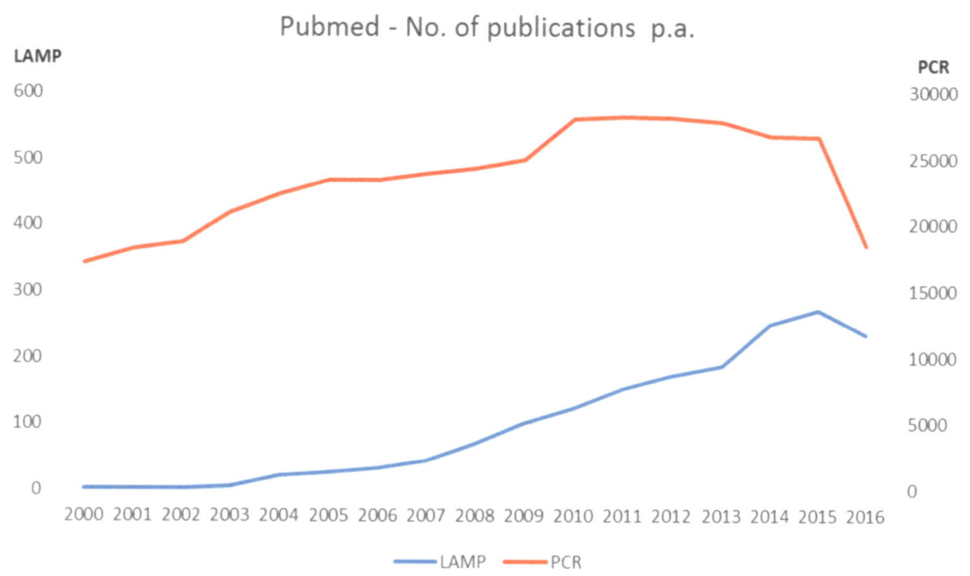

Diagram 1. A comparative graphical representation to illustrate increase in number of publications, LAMP Vs PCR.

3. Loop-mediated isothermal amplification

This review is to introduce the principal concept of a new, advanced, and robust diagnostic method coupled with simplified visualization technique: loop-mediated isothermal amplification (LAMP) with improved sensitivity and specificity for the rapid and reliable detection of *Giardia* DNA.

The LAMP method is a one-step DNA amplification assay performed under isothermal conditions, for 60–120 min using *Bst* polymerase with strand displacement activity and three primer pairs recognizing eight distinct regions within EF-1α (elongation factor-1 alpha) gene for specific detection of *G. duodenalis* (**Figure 1**), producing a considerably high amount of DNA comparable to PCR. The LAMP reaction is carried out in a reaction mixture containing *Bst* polymerase, reaction buffer, primers, DNA template, and a fluorescent dye.

3.1. Primers

LAMP employs two inner primers (FIP and BIP, with typical length of ~40–42 bp), which in turn consists of two parts each and two outer primers (F3, B3 typically length ~ 17–20 bp), which can recognize a total of six distinct regions within the target DNA (see **Figure 1**). The two loop primers employed, forward loop primer (LF) and backward loop primer (LB), were designed to accelerate the amplification reaction and to increase the detection efficiency [37]. In total, six primers recognize eight distinct sites of the target sequence, which can be seen in **Figure 1** indicated as forward (F), backward (B), and complementary (c). In detail, at the 3′ end, the F1c, F2c, and F3c sites are recognized and on the 5′ end, B1, B2, and B3 sites are recognized (**Figure 1, Table 1**). The role of F3 and B3 primers is similar to the ordinary and single domain primers used in PCR amplification. They recognize each one of the six regions resulting in amplification of the entire target DNA sequence.

The most common method for designing LAMP primers is the user-friendly online platform: Primer Explorer V4 software (http://primerexplorer.jp/e) running in Java Runtime Environment, a product of Eiken Chemical Co. Ltd. Additionally, Torres et al. developed an extendable LAMP signature design program called LAMP Assay Versatile Analysis (LAVA) necessary for a high-throughput informatics environment, implemented in Perl script with support modules [38]. And lastly, after the completion of the primer design, specificity of the outer primers (F3 and B3) has to be confirmed with a BLAST search (https://blast.ncbi.nlm.nih.gov/Blast.cgi) in the NCBI database. Several factors are crucial for the performance of LAMP amplification and for optimum primer combinations including GC content, melting temperature (Tm) value, distance between possible primer regions, the stability of primer ends, and ability of possible primers forming secondary structures.

3.2. Mechanism behind the LAMP reaction

The mechanism behind the LAMP reaction involves three major steps: an initial step, a cycling amplification step, and an elongation step.

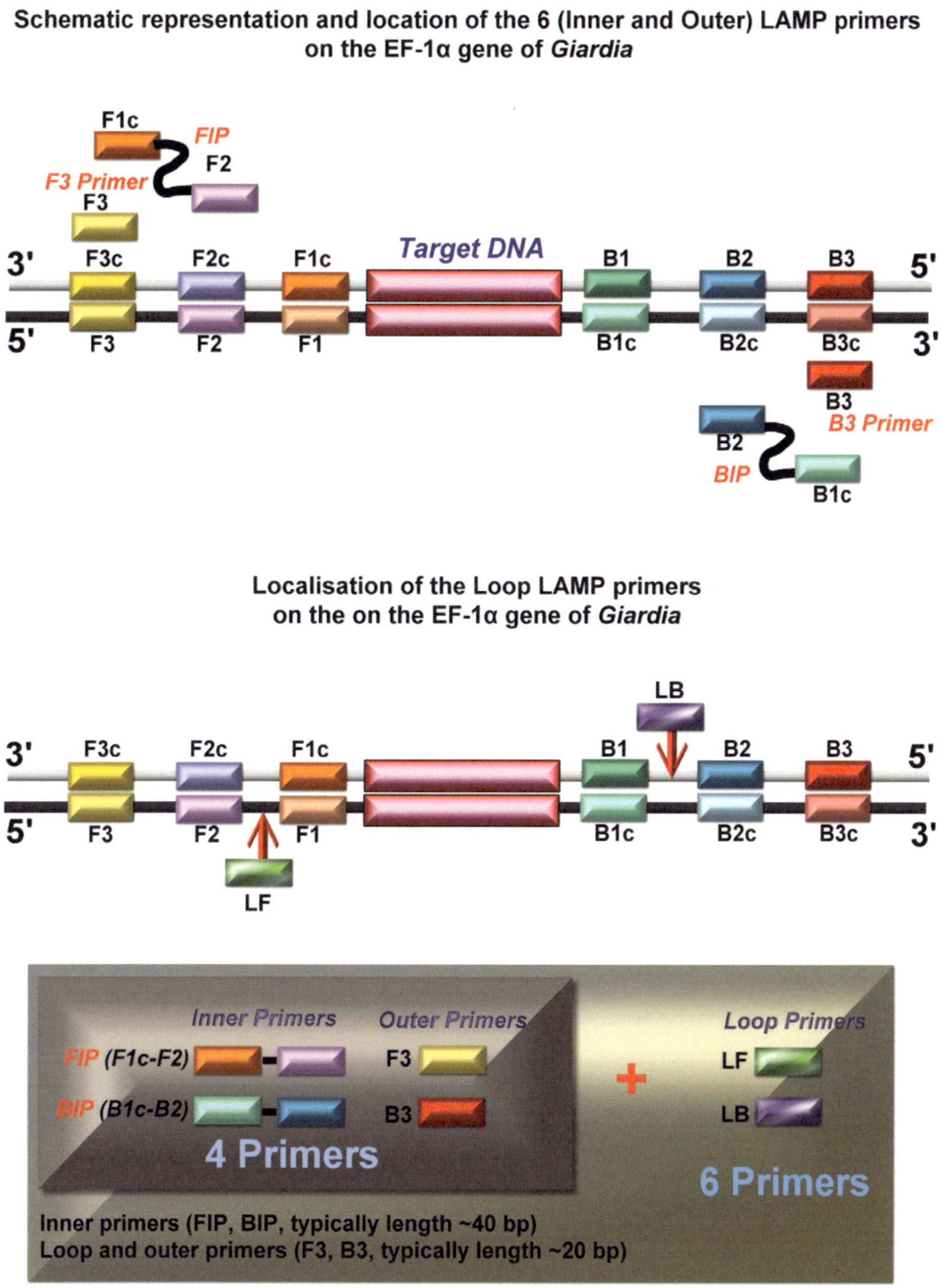

Figure 1. Schematic representation of the three primer pairs recognizing in total eight distinct regions within the EF-1α (elongation factor-1 alpha) gene of *G. duodenalis*.

The simultaneous participation of all six primers is needed for the initial phase production of the starting structure. When the initial phase progresses and during cycling reaction, only the inner primers are used for strand displacement and DNA synthesis. Firstly, one inner FIP

Target	Primer names	Primer sequences	Sequence length	Source/medium	Ref.
Giardia duodenalis EF-1α assemblage B (AF069570)	F3	5′-ATGGACGACGGCCAGG-3′	178 bp	Water, feces, surface water, and sewage samples	[39, 40]
	B3	5′-CCCTCGTACCAGGGCATC-3′			
	FIP	5′-AGCCGATGTTCTTGAGCTGCTT-GTACTCGAAGGAGCGCTACG-3′			
	BIP	5′-GAAGAAGGCCGAGGAGTTCG-TTGTCGGACCTCTCCATGA-3′			
	LB	5′-CTGGACCGGGGACAACA-3′			
	LF	5′-ATCATCTCGCCCTTGATCTCG-3′			
G. duodenalis EF-1α gene	F3	5′- GCCGGGATCTCGAAGGAC-3′	208 bp	Feces pet dogs	[41]
	B3	5′-TCGGGATGTAGTCGAACTCC-3′			
	FIP	5′-T GACCTGGCCGTCGTCCATCTT-GCGACGCTCGCGAACA-3′			
	BIP	5′-G TACTCGAAGGAGCGCTACGAC-GCCTTCTTCCAGCCGATG-3′			
	FLP	5′-GACGGCCAGACGCGCGAG-3′			
	BLP	5′-GCGGAGGGGCTTGTCGGTC-3′			

Table 1. The sequences of the designed primers used for the EF-1α gene of *G. duodenalis* LAMP assays.

http://dx.doi.org/10.5772/intechopen.70804

(BIP) hybrid primer binds to the starting structure, producing the complementary DNA using *Bst* DNA polymerase. F3 (B3) primer binds immediately after the FIP (BIP) primer, displacing the newly synthesized DNA strand and releasing the target DNA or FIP (BIP)-linked complementary DNA strand. Because of the complementarity of F1c and F1 regions, *Bst* polymerase replaces the F3 site of target DNA sequence with F1c of newly released single strand and forms the initial stem loop-loop structure. Similarly and simultaneously, BIP and B3 primers bind to target DNA resulting in formation of single-stranded dumbbell-like starting structure with loops at both ends. The cycling amplification step uses the single-stranded dumbbell-like starting structure as starting material for further amplification in the LAMP reaction. Only the inner primers (FIP and BIP) are used during the cycling amplification step (**Figure 2**).

3.2.1. *Advantages and shortcomings of LAMP assay*

The LAMP assay tenders a spectrum of benefits compared to PCR. Even though PCR is sensitive, it has several intrinsic disadvantages, which limit its successful performance. For instance, the presence of inhibitors and other contents like humic acids interferes with environmental samples resulting in a negative impact on the reaction. PCR operates on the principle of denaturation, annealing, and elongation of DNA with a manifold series of repeated temperature changes. This requires an expensive electronically controlled thermal cycler. LAMP, however, runs under isothermal conditions (without complex variable), which only require a water bath or a heat block. Also, failure or not successful performance of the LAMP reaction due to inhibitors is excluded. Last but not least, the turbidity of positive reaction, which could be seen by naked eyes, obviates further visualization steps, e.g., gel electrophoresis (**Table 2**).

LAMP is considered to be field applicable as the read-out of this method is simplified and is based on naked eye visualization: (a) presence of turbidity in sample, (b) colorimetric change in the case of adding metal-ion indicators, (c) presence of fluorescence by adding DNA-intercalating dyes, and (d) confirmation by gel electrophoresis of the final LAMP products that appear as cauliflower-like structures with multiple loops. Recently, Nzelu et al. established a quick, one-step, single-tube LAMP assay combined with Flinders Technology Associates (FTA) card with pre-added malachite green as a direct sampling tool [39].

3.3. Reaction mixture and reaction conditions

Two reaction mixtures have been reported so far for specific detection of *Giardia duodenalis*. The first protocol uses a buffer containing reagents incorporated in the laboratory, whereas the second protocol uses supplied buffer with *Bst* polymerase. It is recommended to use HPLC-purified primers, if not all, at least FIP and BIP as the primers for purity could be crucial for rapidity and reproducibility of amplification.

The LAMP assay developed for first time during 2009 was carried out in a 25 μl reaction mixture containing 1.6 μM each of FIP and BIP, 0.2 μM each of F3 and B3, 0.8 μM each of LF and LB, 2.8 mM of dNTP, 1.6 M of betaine, 20 mM of Tris-HCl (pH 8.8), 10 mM of KCl, 10 mM

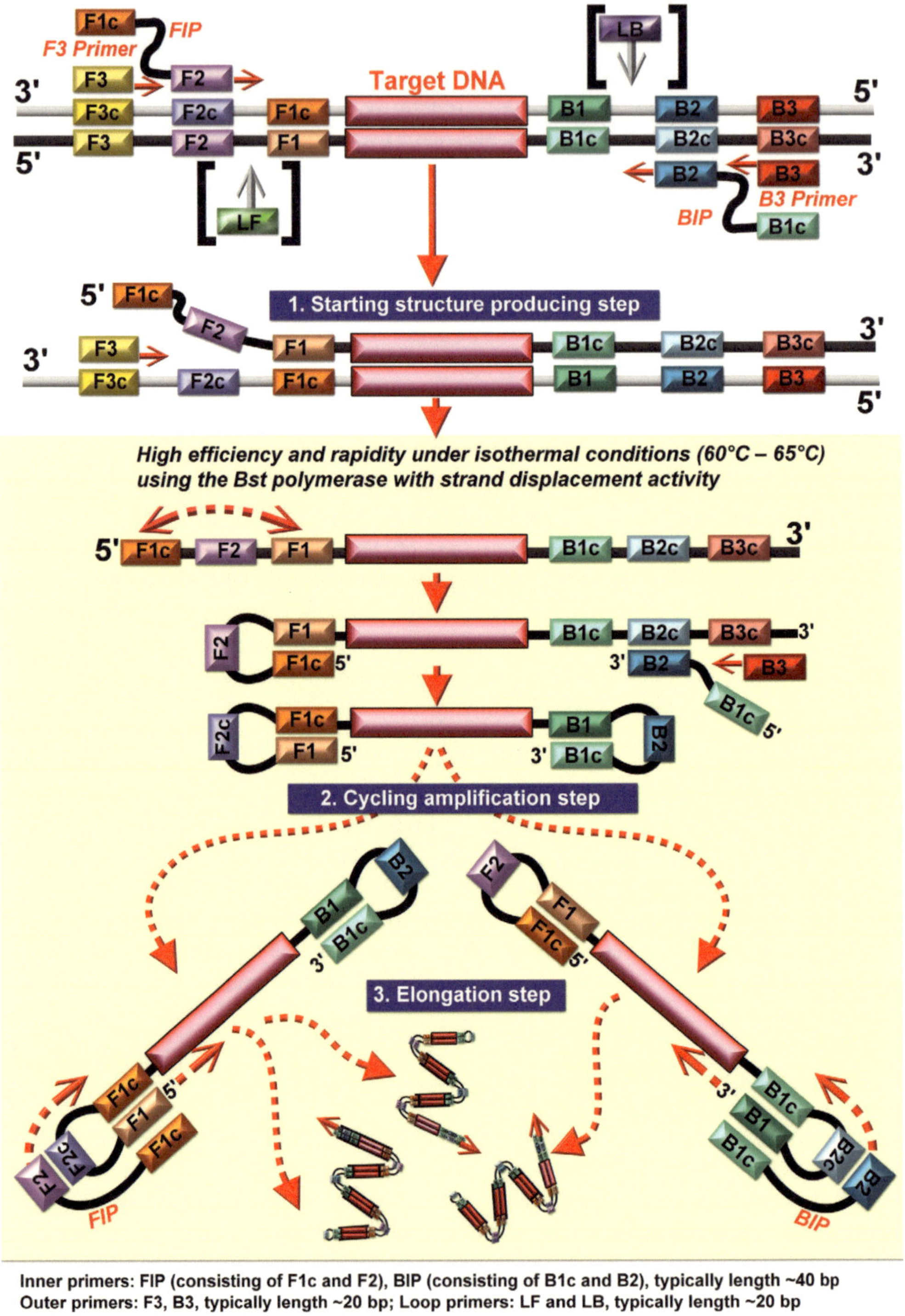

Figure 2. Simplified schematic representation of the major steps in the LAMP method and localization of the eight LAMP primers on target DNA sequence for specific amplification of EF1α gene of *G. duodenalis*.

	PCR	LAMP
Advantages	Sensitive	• Sensitive (10- to100-fold) • Specific (designed to amplify six or eight different regions of the target gene) • Easy • Rapid • Cost effective • Quick
	Genotyping of the amplified product	Isothermal conditions
		Polymerase with strand displacement activity and no need of heat denaturation of the double-stranded DNA products
	Amplification in thermal cycler, variation in temperature	Amplification in water bath or a heat block Constant temperature Simple and cost-effective equipment
	Interpretation of results in gel electrophoresis	• Interpretation of results by naked eye • Presence or absence of turbidity through production of white precipitate of magnesium pyrophosphate • Colorimetric change after the addition of HNB, malachite green or SYBR green, SYTO-82, SYTO-84, and SYTOX Orange • Fluorescence detection under UV light • Gel electrophoresis • Real-time monitoring turbidimeter • Field applicable
Deficiencies	Only DNA fragments Sequencing of the amplified reaction product	Only DNA fragments Sequencing: possible with limitations
	Time consuming	Multiplex-LAMP difficult
	Inhibitors	Crosscontamination
	Expensive thermal cycler	Need of further progress

Table 2. Advantages and shortcomings of LAMP assay in comparison to PCR.

of $(NH_4)_2SO_4$, 16 mM of $MgSO_4$, 0.2% Tween 20, and the DNA template (2 μl). The reaction mixture was heated at 95°C for 2 min and then chilled on ice. Next, 8 U *Bst* DNA polymerase large fragments were added followed by incubation at 63°C for 120 min and heating at 80°C for 7 min to terminate the reaction [40]. In a consecutive report, the primer concentration was as follows: 40 pmol each of FIP and BIP primers, 20 pmol each of LF and LB primers, and 5 pmol each of F3 and B3 primers [41, 42].

The second protocol was developed in 2013 wherein the LAMP assay was carried out in a 25 μl reaction mixture containing 10× *Bst*-DNA polymerase buffer, 1.6 M betaine, 2.5 mM each deoxynucleotide triphosphates, 8 mM $MgSO_4$, 0.2 μM each F3 and B3 primers, 1.6 μM each FIP and BIP, 0.8 μM each loop-F and loop-B, 8 U *Bst* DNA polymerase 1 μl of 10,000× concentrated SYBR Green I, and template DNA (2 μl). In this case, the mixture was incubated at 63°C for 60 min and then heated at 80°C for 10 min [43].

3.4. Specificity assessment of the LAMP assay

The specificity of both aforementioned protocols was determined by testing DNA derived from *G. duodenalis* cysts and from phylogenetically related protozoan parasites. This includes *Cryptosporidium parvum, Trypanosoma brucei, Theileria parva, Toxoplasma gondii, Babesia bovis,* plankton biomass, and *G. duodenalis* assemblages A and B for the first protocol [40] and *Toxoplasma gondii, Neospora caninum, Cryptosporidium parvum, Eimeria tenella, and G. duodenalis* for the second protocol [43].

3.5. Sensitivity assessment of the LAMP assay

The sensitivity was assessed using 10-fold dilutions of genomic DNA, and the results demonstrated that LAMP successfully amplified 0.548 pg. DNA/tube (corresponding to ~four cysts) for *G. duodenalis* assemblage B and 0.8 pg. DNA/tube (corresponding to ~six cysts) for *G. duodenalis* assemblage A for the first protocol [40]. The detection limit for the second protocol was 10^{-4} ng/μl (0.1 pg/μl) and 10 times more sensitive than the PCR assay [43].

3.6. Sample collection and purification methods applied in combination with the LAMP

During the development of LAMP methodology for the first time, Plutzer et al. applied it in 10 surface water samples and 15 sewage samples, all collected between 2004 and 2007 in Hungary and previously tested and identified as positive using ImmunoFluorescence Test (IFT) [40, 44]. They also used 10 human fecal samples from Hungarian human patients reported with gastroenteritis in 2007. All samples were amplified by PCRs targeting 18S rRNA [45], glutamate dehydrogenase (GDH) genes [46], triosephosphate isomerase (TPI) gene [47], and EF-1α LAMP. They found that 33 of 35 (94%) environmental and fecal samples were positive for *G. duodenalis* according to one or more of applied techniques. Here, we would like to emphasize that *G. duodenalis*-specific LAMP-amplified DNA was positive in 24 of 35 predefined positive samples, while 23 were positive for 18S rRNA, 15 for GDH, and only 3 for TPI (**Table 3**).

On a more extensive work, the same authors examined 132 aquatic bird fecal samples, collected from February to March 2008 in Hungary [41]. The fecal samples were placed in tubes using polystyrene spatulas and were homogenized in 50 ml of distilled water followed by sieving through 0.1 -mm pore size sieve. After centrifugation, 50 μl of fecal samples were subject to IFT and 2-(4-amidinophenyl)-6-indolecarbamidine dihydrochloride [DAPI], whereas the remaining part underwent DNA extraction and was subject to 18S rRNA PCR and EF-1α LAMP. Altogether four fecal samples were positive for *Giardia* by IFT, five by PCR, and five by LAMP. Interestingly, *Giardia* in common was identified only in one sample with IFT. In none of the other cases was there a simultaneous/overlap identification of *Giardia* using LAMP or PCR. It is worth to mention that the quality of extracted DNA was assessed in this case with

Matrix/no. of investigated samples	Collection and purification methods	Investigated volume	DNA extraction	PCR target gene	LAMP target gene	Ref.
Surface water ($n = 10$)	Chemical flocculation or membrane filtration	10–20 L	QIAmp Mini Kit	18S rRNA GDH, TPI	EF-1α[1]	[40]
Sewage water ($n = 15$)			QIAmp Stool Kit*			
Fecal samples ($n = 10$)	IMS	10 ml	QIAmp Mini Kit and*			
Fecal samples ($n = 132$)	Polystyrene spatulas and sieved through 0.1 mm pore size sieve	homogenized in 50 ml distilled water	QIAamp Stool Kit	18 S rRNA	EF-1α[1]	[41]
Drinking water ($n = 27$)	ARAD microfiber filtration, centrifugation, and vacuum filtration through 3 μm ISOPORE membrane	10–1000 L	QIAmp Mini kit*,**	—	EF-1α[1]	[42]
River water ($n = 20$)	Membrane filtration (diameter 142 mm), pore size 1.2 μm and sucrose flotation	10 L	QIAamp Mini Kit*	GDH	EF-1α[1]	[48]
Fecal samples ($n = 39$)	Sieved through four layers of gauze and centrifugation	5 gr	QIAamp DNA Stool Mini Kit	bg	EF-1α[1]	[49]
Fecal samples ($n = 72$)	flotation technique with saturated zinc sulfate and purification by sucrose gradient	—	QIAamp DNA Stool Mini Kit	Ef-1a (performed with the outer primers B3 and F3)	EF-1α	[43]
WWTPs water ($n = 138$)	$Al_2(SO_4)_3$ Aluminum sulfate flocculation, and sucrose centrifugation	5 L for influent and 2 L for effluent	QIAamp Mini Kit	16S rRNA	EF-1α[1]	[50]
• Surface water, • Groundwater, raw and drinking water	microfiber filtration (ARAD and Sheather's sugar solution	(a) Up to 400 L (b) Up to 6300 L				
Environmental water samples ($n = 420$)	$Al_2(SO_4)_3$ flocculation and sucrose flotation	10 L	QIAamp DNA Mini Kit	(SSU)rRNA, GDH	EF-1α[1]	[51]
Drinking water samples ($n = 120$)						

[1]Primers used according to [40].

*Modification of the manufacturer protocol: addition of ten 10-min freeze-thaw cycles after resuspension in lysis solution.

**Elution with 32-μl LAMP buffer [40 mmol l^{-1} Tris-HCL, 20 mmol l^{-1} KCl, 16 mmol l^{-1} $MgSO_4$, 20 mmol l^{-1} $(NH_4)_2SO_4$, 0.2 v/v % Tween 20, 16 mol l^{-1} betaine, and 28 mmol l^{-1} each deoxynucleoside triphosphate].

-: not reported; bg: beta-giardin; IMS: Immunomagnetic separation (Dynabeads GC-Combo kit, Dynal Biotech); GDH: glutamate dehydrogenase gene; WWTPs: wastewater treatment plants.

Table 3. Results on evaluation studies of the sample collection and purification methods applied in combination with the LAMP in different matrices.

the inclusion of internal controls and identified that their amplification was unsuccessful in 17% of the samples of which nine were positive for *Giardia* by LAMP [41].

To clarify the role of sample inhibitors, 27 drinking water samples of 10–1000 L were collected over a 24-h time period using the ARAD filtration system and were spiked with 100 *G. duodenalis* cysts. The genomic DNA from the samples (water spiked with *G. duodenalis* cysts) was extracted and then EF-1α LAMP was performed. The results showed that LAMP reaction was not affected by inhibitors in any of the samples tested [42].

In total, 10 L Iranian surface water samples from two rivers, collected over a time period of 12 months, were filtered using 142 mm membrane filters and were comparably investigated using IFT, PCR targeting the GDH gene, and LAMP targeting the EF-1α gene. Prior to genomic DNA extraction using the QIAamp Mini Kit, all river water samples were purified through sucrose flotation. The prevalence of *G. duodenalis* cysts was 13 out of 20 water samples by IFT, 10 out of 20 by the GDH gene PCR, and 8 out of 20 by EF-1α gene LAMP assay [48]. Notably in this study, the recovery rate of the protocol was assessed in 5 L water samples, seeded with 5 and 10 cyst/L, and they reported that the mean recovery rate for *Giardia* cysts in the seeded water samples was 18% and all of them tested positive by PCR and LAMP analysis.

During 2015, Çiçek and Şakru used effectively *Giardia* LAMP assay in 39 human fecal samples obtained from Turkey [49]. They primarily screened the patient's fecal material microscopically in native and stained with lugol iodine method to determine the cyst density. After that, samples were subject to DNA extraction using QIAamp DNA Stool Mini Kit and tested for EF-1α gene using LAMP for *Giardia* and beta-giardin (bg) PCR. EF-1α gene LAMP and bg gene region PCR for detection of *G. intestinalis* were found positive in 32 (82%) and 19 (48.7%) of the cases, respectively. Interestingly, the authors stated a significant difference between patients with higher cyst density and lower cyst density ($p = 0.0001$) through the PCR positivity rate [49].

An existing literature documents the performance of EF-1α gene LAMP for detection of *Giardia* in environmental water samples in Germany [50]. The investigators of this study examined a wide palette of different water types and compared the effectiveness of three detection methods: IFT, PCR, and LAMP. A total number of 185 samples originated from influent and effluent wastewater treatment plants (WWTPs), surface waters, a recreational area, groundwater, untreated water from a drinking water plant, and tap water were analyzed during the period from July 2009 to January 2011. For the extraction of the genomic DNA of all sample types, QIAamp Mini Kit was used [50]. All the samples were investigated by three detection assays: IFT, 16S rRNA by PCR, and EF-1α gene by LAMP. The comparison of the three methods indicated better results with IFT compared with the DNA-based assays, among which the LAMP assay was more sensitive than the applied PCR for detection of *Giardia*. The ranking results were as follows: IFA over LAMP and LAMP over nested PCR (56.8 > 42.7 > 33.5%, respectively). Despite nonconcordance of the methods resulting from statistical calculations, the authors outlined differences considering analytical steps such as sample preparation, DNA extraction, and analytical targets. A further explanation closely related to the variable detection capabilities of the assays according to authors is that the samples might contain *G. duodenalis* assemblages other than A and B, which might not be detected by LAMP but may be detected by PCR and/or IFT. The authors in this case speculated a little further over data interpretation and concluded that another unambiguous factor for the superiority of IFT over the other methods is also possible as IFT detects at the taxonomic level of respective *Giardia* genera and the assemblages cannot be discriminated by this method.

Between 2012 and 2014, Koloren et al. collected 420 environmental and 120 drinking water samples from Turkey [51]. All samples were collected by $Al_2(SO_4)_3$ flocculation and were purified by sucrose flotation technique. DNA isolation was conducted in the purified samples according to QIAamp DNA Mini Kit protocol, and they investigated all samples using EF-1α gene LAMP, small subunit (SSU) rRNA, and GDH PCR. A total of 141 (58.7%), 125 (52.1%), and 120 (50%) were identified positive by each of the aforementioned methods, respectively [51].

Li et al. developed an alternative protocol, including new primer pairs detecting the EF-1α gene of *Giardia*, with potential application for clinical diagnosis of *G. lamblia* from dogs' feces. They collected feces from dogs and processed them by flotation technique with saturated zinc sulfate and purification by sucrose gradient solution. To obtain the genomic DNA template, purified cysts from all fecal samples were subject to QIAamp DNA Stool Mini Kit. The results of microscopy, PCR (performed with the outer primers B3 and F3 of the LAMP assay), and EF-1α gene LAMP for *Giardia* were compared and the results showed that 5 (6.9%) of the 72 dog fecal samples tested positive by microscopy, and 7 (9.7%) and 8 (11.1%) tested positive by PCR and LAMP, respectively [43].

Thoughtfully, we are describing the results of an investigation of Nago et al. (unfortunately, whose contents, preparation steps, and details of the full text are not at our disposal) [52]. They reported that they developed a LAMP assay capable of detecting 3.12×10^{-1} *G. lamblia* cysts per reaction in spiked fecal specimens. Out of the 19 spiked samples, 16 (84%) were successfully amplified by LAMP assay and resulted in positive readings. Furthermore, they attempted to ascertain the negative reaction result in three fecal samples, which is likely due to inhibition. For this, they investigated two specific parameters: dilutions of extracted DNA and addition of bovine serum albumin (BSA) to the LAMP reaction mixture. This modification seemed to yield positive results and to have positive effect on the occurrence of false-negative readings.

3.7. The current momentum toward LAMP

G. duodenalis is one of the most prominent waterborne parasite worldwide and causative agent for several outbreaks in developing, developed, and industrialized countries with fatal consequences, mostly affecting the weakest of the population [12, 13]. The lack of sanitation and health care in Third World nations where malnutrition due to scarcity of food is common leads to highest prevalence of giardiasis in the population. As is often the case, the most vulnerable population groups are also the worst affected: children under the age of 5 years, elderly, and immunocompromised people. Particularly, the mortality rate is correspondingly and shatteringly high among these groups. As a result, scientists and politicians should be encouraged to counteract this dilemma at all levels. Key measures not only include the establishment of appropriate hygiene measures and sanitary facilities and access to clean water but also, or in particular, the setting up of surveillance systems and monitoring programs.

As is often said, prevention is better than cure. However, scanning the objective slides with a microscope is time consuming and exhausting. Cysts could be covered in debris or if at all when available for examination, each cyst will have to be checked for different morphological characteristics, and therefore, skilled technicians are needed. Due to the visualization difficulties of microscopic readings from samples, significant progress has been made in molecular methods such as PCR and PCR-RFLP aiming at proper characterization of *G. duodenalis* into its different assemblages and subassemblages. Therefore, researchers are frequently confronted with the challenge of defining new methods, specific for rapid and accurate diagnosis and for tracking the source of contamination. This is necessary in order to provide efficient treatment and prevent grievance. Even though we have managed to overcome some of the upcoming obstacles, the presence of inhibitors, low sensitivity of molecular methods, and lack of inter- and in some cases intralaboratory standardization in PCR methods are the main reasons that urge scientists to develop further methods.

Water is worth protecting and is the most important nutrient. Contamination of water by *G. duodenalis* is a health risk to all of us. Infective stages of *Giardia* species are able to persist in the aquatic environment for months, which is also the major route of infection. The fast and reliable detection of the parasites and ability to trace its origin can curb the occurrence of larger outbreaks or epidemics premature or better, even avoid one.

With this chapter, we would like to emphasize how effective the innovative LAMP process is. It is worth to be presented to a large specialist audience: one because it offers many advantages over other detection methods and secondly as it is very efficient and easy to carry out without the need for expensive equipment. Moreover, in this case, it is irrelevant that test matrix available for analysis. The detection is easy in stool and tissue samples as well as in environmental samples, mud, and water.

The chapter summarizes all relevant information on the detection of *G. duodenalis* with the LAMP procedure and gives a comprehensive overview of the current state of the art. This is a collection of all available protocols related to the development and application of a simple field-usable method that can meet the needs for a quicker and objective readout for the diagnosis of giardiasis in water and feces. The LAMP assay is ranked among the most accurate molecular tools thanks to its high diagnostic sensitivity and specificity. The future utility of a simple portable device (tube scanner) in which both the amplification platform (heating block) and fluorescent detection unit for end point use (with the ability to acquire real time data) has been envisioned to be combined into a single unit for LAMP assay for the detection of *Giardia* infections.

At present, LAMP is entering the ranks of the recognized detection methods among the World Health Organization (WHO) collaborating centers on foodborne trematode infections. This has been achieved mainly after the reported diagnosis of *Opisthorchis viverrini* infection in stool samples by the use of the LAMP technique [53]. The establishment and the use of a commercial LAMP assay (TB-LAMP) for the detection of tuberculosis was the subject of the expert group meeting organized by the WHO in Geneva in May 2013, and they certified LAMP as a potential diagnostic test. During the last year, CDC-UGA had financially supported the development of RealAmp-LAMP platform for the accurate detection of *Plasmodium vivax* infections [54]. The LAMP is considered as a technology under development with potential for future application and is currently undergoing large-scale evaluation by the Foundation for Innovative new Diagnostics (FIND) [55] and Centers for Disease Control (CDC) [55]. The proposed method can be expanded to be a quick and specific alternative screening technique for other life-threatening pathogens such as Ebola virus, human papilloma virus (HPV), human immunodeficiency virus (HIV), hepatitis C, etc. Moreover, in case of outbreaks, it could help prevent progression to active disease through early detection in saliva and examine the distribution of pathogens in different body fluids during infectious and noninfectious phases.

The establishment of surveillance activities is the most important step for health care professionals in prevention and in case of outbreaks tracking the source of contamination as fast as possible. Therefore, we advocate for LAMP as a suitable tool, in which given this expense and the large number of ongoing projects addressing, there is clearly a need for the development of a fast, economic assay, and user-friendly approach to detect *G. duodenalis* by fastest possible processing.

Author details

Carmen Gallas-Lindemann[1], Poornima Sureshkumar[2], Michael J. Noack[3] and Isaia Sotiriadou[3]*

*Address all correspondence to: isaia.sotiriadou@uk-koeln.de

1 Linksniederrheinische Entwässerungs-Genossenschaft, Kamp-Lintfort, Germany

2 Center of Physiology and Pathophysiology, Institute of Neurophysiology, University of Cologne, Cologne, Germany

3 Centre of Dental Medicine, Policlinic of Operative Dentistry and Periodontology, University of Cologne, Cologne, Germany

References

[1] Cavalier-Smith T. Protist phylogeny and the high-level classification of protozoa. European Journal of Protistology. 2003;**39**(4):338-348

[2] Morrison HG, McArthur AG, Gillin FD, Aley SB, Adam RD, Olsen GJ, et al. Genomic minimalism in the early diverging intestinal parasite *Giardia lamblia*. Science. 2007; **317**(5846):1921-1926 Epub 29 September 2007

[3] Ansari MAR. An epitome on the present state of our knowledge of the parasitic duodenal flagellate of man-*Giardia intestinalis* (Lambl, 1859). Pakistan Journal of Health. 1954;**4**:131-158

[4] Mehlhorn H, Piekarski G. Grundriß der Parasitenkunde: Parasiten des Menschen und der Nutztiere. Akad. Vlg., Hdg.; Auflage: 5., überarb. A. 1998

[5] Heyworth MF. *Giardia duodenalis* genetic assemblages and hosts. Parasite. 2016;**23**:13 Epub 18 March 2016

[6] Lasek-Nesselquist E, Welch DM, Sogin ML. The identification of a new *Giardia duodenalis* assemblage in marine vertebrates and a preliminary analysis of *G. duodenalis* population biology in marine systems. International Journal for Parasitology. 2010;**40**(9):1063-1074 Epub 7 April 2010

[7] Plutzer J, Ongerth J, Karanis P. *Giardia* taxonomy, phylogeny and epidemiology: Facts and open questions. International Journal of Hygiene and Environmental Health. 2010;**213**(5):321-333 Epub 14 July 2010

[8] Feng Y, Xiao L. Zoonotic potential and molecular epidemiology of *Giardia* species and giardiasis. Clinical Microbiology Reviews. 2011;**24**(1):110-140 Epub 15 January 2011

[9] Huang DB, White AC. An updated review on *Cryptosporidium* and *Giardia*. Gastroenterology Clinics of North America. 2006;**35**(2):291-314, viii Epub 2 August 2006

[10] Erickson MC, Ortega YR. Inactivation of protozoan parasites in food, water, and environmental systems. Journal of Food Protection. 2006;**69**(11):2786-2808 Epub 1 December 2006

[11] Rendtorff RC, Holt CJ. The experimental transmission of human intestinal protozoan parasites. IV. Attempts to transmit *Endamoeba coli* and *Giardia lamblia* cysts by water. American Journal of Hygiene. 1954;**60**(3):327-338 Epub 1 November 1954

[12] Baldursson S, Karanis P. Waterborne transmission of protozoan parasites: Review of worldwide outbreaks—An update 2004-2010. Water Research. 2011;**45**(20):6603-6614 Epub 4 November 2011

[13] Efstratiou A, Ongerth JE, Karanis P. Waterborne transmission of protozoan parasites: Review of worldwide outbreaks—An update 2011-2016. Water Research. 2017;**114**:14-22 Epub 20 February 2017

[14] Giangaspero A, Berrilli F, Brandonisio O. *Giardia* and *Cryptosporidium* and public health: The epidemiological scenario from the Italian perspective. Parasitology Research. 2007;**101**(5):1169-1182 Epub 27 June 2007

[15] Daryani A, Sharif M, Meigouni M, Mahmoudi FB, Rafiei A, Gholami S, et al. Prevalence of intestinal parasites and profile of CD4+ counts in HIV+/AIDS people in north of Iran, 2007-2008. Pakistan Journal of Biological Sciences. 2009;**12**(18):1277-1281 Epub 14 April 2010

[16] Eckmann L. Mucosal defences against *Giardia*. Parasite Immunology. 2003;**25**(5):259-270 Epub 13 September 2003

[17] Sahagun J, Clavel A, Goni P, Seral C, Llorente MT, Castillo FJ, et al. Correlation between the presence of symptoms and the *Giardia duodenalis* genotype. European Journal of Clinical Microbiology & Infectious Diseases: Official publication of the European Society of Clinical Microbiology. 2008;**27**(1):81-83 Epub 19 October 2007

[18] Nash TE, Herrington DA, Losonsky GA, Levine MM. Experimental human infections with *Giardia lamblia*. The Journal of Infectious Diseases. 1987;**156**(6):974-984 Epub 1 December 1987

[19] Nash TE, Herrington DA, Levine MM, Conrad JT, Merritt JW Jr. Antigenic variation of *Giardia lamblia* in experimental human infections. Journal of Immunology. 1990;**144**(11):4362-4369 Epub 1 June 1990

[20] Robertson LJ, Hanevik K, Escobedo AA, Morch K, Langeland N. Giardiasis—Why do the symptoms sometimes never stop? Trends in Parasitology. 2010;**26**(2):75-82 Epub 9 January 2010

[21] Escobedo AA, Almirall P, Robertson LJ, Franco RM, Hanevik K, Morch K, et al. Giardiasis: The ever-present threat of a neglected disease. Infectious Disorders Drug Targets. 2010;**10**(5):329-348 Epub 13 August 2010

[22] Rossignol JF. *Cryptosporidium* and *Giardia*: Treatment options and prospects for new drugs. Experimental Parasitology. 2010;**124**(1):45-53 Epub 28 July 2009

[23] Yang K, LeJeune J, Alsdorf D, Lu B, Shum CK, Liang S. Global distribution of outbreaks of water-associated infectious diseases. PLoS Neglected Tropical Diseases. 2012;**6**(2):e148e3 Epub 22 February 2012

[24] Dixon B, Parrington L, Cook A, Pollari F, Farber J. Detection of *Cyclospora*, *Cryptosporidium*, and *Giardia* in ready-to-eat packaged leafy greens in Ontario, Canada. Journal of Food Protection. 2013;**76**(2):307-313 Epub 26 February 2013

[25] Budu-Amoako E, Greenwood SJ, Dixon BR, Barkema HW, McClure JT. Foodborne illness associated with *Cryptosporidium* and *Giardia* from livestock. Journal of Food Protection. 2011;**74**(11):1944-1955 Epub 8 November 2011

[26] Mateo M, Montoya A, Bailo B, Saugar JM, Aguilera M, Fuentes I, et al. Detection and molecular characterization of *Giardia duodenalis* in children attending day care centers in Majadahonda, Madrid, Central Spain. Medicine. 2014;**93**(15):e75 Epub 3 October 2014

[27] Steketee RW, Reid S, Cheng T, Stoebig JS, Harrington RG, Davis JP. Recurrent outbreaks of giardiasis in a child day care center, Wisconsin. American Journal of Public Health. 1989;**79**(4):485-490 Epub 1 April 1989

[28] Sagnuankiat S, Wanichsuwan M, Bhunnachet E, Jungarat N, Panraksa K, Komalamisra C, et al. Health status of immigrant children and environmental survey of child daycare centers in Samut Sakhon Province, Thailand. Journal of Immigrant and Minority Health. 2016;**18**(1):21-27 Epub 17 December 2014

[29] Gallas-Lindemann C, Sotiriadou I, Plutzer J, Karanis P. Prevalence and distribution of *Cryptosporidium* and *Giardia* in wastewater and the surface, drinking and ground waters in the lower Rhine, Germany. Epidemiology and Infection. 2013;**141**(1):9-21 Epub 27 September 2012

[30] Robert Koch-Institut. Aktuelle daten und informationen zu infektionskrankheiten und public health. 16 März 2017/Nr. 11/12 http://www.rki.de/DE/Content/Infekt/EpidBull/Archiv/2017/Ausgaben/11-12_17.pdf?__blob=publicationFile

[31] Connor BA. Chronic diarrhea in travelers. Current Infectious Disease Reports. 2013;**15**(3):203-210 Epub 28 March 2013

[32] Ignatius R, Gahutu JB, Klotz C, Steininger C, Shyirambere C, Lyng M, et al. High prevalence of *Giardia duodenalis* assemblage B infection and association with underweight in Rwandan children. PLoS Neglected Tropical Diseases. 2012;**6**(6):e1677 Epub 22 June 2012

[33] Staudacher O, Heimer J, Steiner F, Kayonga Y, Havugimana JM, Ignatius R, et al. Soil-transmitted helminths in southern highland Rwanda: Associated factors and effectiveness of school-based preventive chemotherapy. Tropical Medicine & International Health. 2014;**19**(7):812-824 Epub 23 April 2014

[34] UNHCfRUGtFdi. 2015. http://www.unhcr.org/576408cd7. [Accessed: March 2017]

[35] Theuring S, Friedrich-Janicke B, Portner K, Trebesch I, Durst A, Dieckmann S, et al. Screening for infectious diseases among unaccompanied minor refugees in Berlin, 2014-2015. European Journal of Epidemiology. 2016;**31**(7):707-710 Epub 28 July 2016

[36] Notomi T, Okayama H, Masubuchi H, Yonekawa T, Watanabe K, Amino N, et al. Loop-mediated isothermal amplification of DNA. Nucleic Acids Research. 2000;**28**(12):E63 Epub 28 June 2000

[37] Nagamine K, Hase T, Notomi T. Accelerated reaction by loop-mediated isothermal amplification using loop primers. Molecular and Cellular Probes. 2002;**16**(3):223-229 Epub 30 July 2002

[38] Torres C, Vitalis EA, Baker BR, Gardner SN, Torres MW, Dzenitis JM. LAVA: An open-source approach to designing LAMP (loop-mediated isothermal amplification) DNA signatures. BMC Bioinformatics. 2011;**12**:240 Epub 18 June 2011

[39] Nzelu CO, Caceres AG, Guerrero-Quincho S, Tineo-Villafuerte E, Rodriquez-Delfin L, Mimori T, et al. A rapid molecular diagnosis of cutaneous leishmaniasis by colorimetric malachite green-loop-mediated isothermal amplification (LAMP) combined with an FTA card as a direct sampling tool. Acta Tropica. 2016;**153**:116-119 Epub 31 October 2015

[40] Plutzer J, Karanis P. Rapid identification of *Giardia duodenalis* by loop-mediated isothermal amplification (LAMP) from faecal and environmental samples and comparative findings by PCR and real-time PCR methods. Parasitology Research. 2009;**104**(6):1527-1533 Epub 17 March 2009

[41] Plutzer J, Tomor B. The role of aquatic birds in the environmental dissemination of human pathogenic *Giardia duodenalis* cysts and *Cryptosporidium* oocysts in Hungary. Parasitology International. 2009;**58**(3):227-231 Epub 19 May 2009

[42] Plutzer J, Torokne A, Karanis P. Combination of ARAD microfibre filtration and LAMP methodology for simple, rapid and cost-effective detection of human pathogenic Giardia

duodenalis and *Cryptosporidium* spp. in drinking water. Letters in Applied Microbiology. 2010;**50**(1):82-88 Epub 10 November 2009

[43] Li J, Wang P, Zhang A, Zhang P, Alsarakibi M, Li G. Sensitive and rapid detection of *Giardia lamblia* infection in pet dogs using loop-mediated isothermal amplification. The Korean Journal of Parasitology. 2013;**51**(2):237-241 Epub 28 May 2013

[44] Plutzer J, Karanis P, Domokos K, Torokne A, Marialigeti K. Detection and characterisation of *Giardia* and *Cryptosporidium* in Hungarian raw, surface and sewage water samples by IFT, PCR and sequence analysis of the SSUrRNA and GDH genes. International Journal of Hygiene and Environmental Health. 2008;**211**(5-6):524-533 Epub 14 June 2008

[45] Appelbee AJ, Frederick LM, Heitman TL, Olson ME. Prevalence and genotyping of *Giardia duodenalis* from beef calves in Alberta, Canada. Veterinary Parasitology. 2003;**112**(4):289-294 Epub 8 March 2003

[46] Read CM, Monis PT, Thompson RC. Discrimination of all genotypes of *Giardia duodenalis* at the glutamate dehydrogenase locus using PCR-RFLP. Infection, Genetics and Evolution: Journal of Molecular Epidemiology and Evolutionary Genetics in Infectious Diseases. 2004;**4**(2):125-130 Epub 26 May 2004

[47] Amar CF, Dear PH, McLauchlin J. Detection and genotyping by real-time PCR/RFLP analyses of *Giardia duodenalis* from human faeces. Journal of Medical Microbiology. 2003;**52**(Pt 8):681-683 Epub 18 July 2003

[48] Mahmoudi MR, Kazemi B, Mohammadiha A, Mirzaei A, Karanis P. Detection of *Cryptosporidium* and *Giardia* (oo)cysts by IFA, PCR and LAMP in surface water from Rasht, Iran. Transactions of the Royal Society of Tropical Medicine and Hygiene. 2013;**107**(8):511-517 Epub 6 June 2013

[49] Cicek C, Sakru N. Trakya Bolgesi'ndeki *Giardia intestinalis* izolatlarinin genotiplendirilmesi [Genotyping of *Giardia* Intestinalis isolates in the Thrace region, Turkey]. Mikrobiyoloji bulteni. 2015;**49**(4):576-585 Epub 10 December 2015

[50] Gallas-Lindemann C, Sotiriadou I, Plutzer J, Noack MJ, Mahmoudi MR, Karanis P. *Giardia* and *Cryptosporidium* spp. dissemination during wastewater treatment and comparative detection via immunofluorescence assay (IFA), nested polymerase chain reaction (nested PCR) and loop mediated isothermal amplification (LAMP). Acta Tropica. 2016;**158**:43-51 Epub 18 February 2016

[51] Koloren Z, Seferoglu O, Karanis P. Occurency of *Giardia duodenalis* assemblages in river water sources of Black Sea, Turkey. Acta Tropica. 2016;**164**:337-344

[52] Nago TT, Tokashiki YT, Kisanuki K, Nakasone I, Yamane N. Laboratory-based evaluation of loop-mediated isothermal amplification (LAMP) to detect *Cryptosporidium* oocyst and *Giardia lamblia* cyst in stool specimens. Rinsho byori The Japanese Journal of Clinical Pathology. 2010;**58**(8):765-771 Epub 24 September 2010

[53] Arimatsu Y, Kaewkes S, Laha T, Sripa B. Specific diagnosis of *Opisthorchis viverrini* using loop-mediated isothermal amplification (LAMP) targeting parasite microsatellites. Acta Tropica. 2015;**141**(Pt B):368-371 Epub 1 October 2014

[54] Patel JC, Oberstaller J, Xayavong M, Narayanan J, DeBarry JD, Srinivasamoorthy G, et al. Real-time loop-mediated isothermal amplification (RealAmp) for the species-specific identification of *Plasmodium vivax*. PLoS One. 2013;**8**(1):e54986 Epub 26 January 2013

[55] Cuevas LE. The urgent need for new diagnostics for symptomatic tuberculosis in children. Indian Journal of Pediatrics. 2011;**78**(4):449-455 Epub 29 December 2010

Section 3

Treatment, Prevention and Public Health

Chapter 8

Pharmacological Treatment of Giardiasis

Víctor Manuel Molina Díaz

Additional information is available at the end of the chapter

http://dx.doi.org/10.5772/intechopen.71803

Abstract

Giardiasis is a disease caused for a myoflagellate protozoan known as *Giardia duodenalis*, of which varieties have been described and whose morphological characteristics are identical to other species such as *G. lamblia* and *G. intestinalis*; considered for various authors as the same species, this protozoan parasites several domestic species including man, but has important relevance in the canine and feline species, due to their zoonotic potential. In recent years, the number of cases of canine and feline giardiasis has increased, not only because it is treated of a cosmopolitan parasite, which is closely related to unsanitary conditions, but also because the conventional treatments for its control and eradication have shown resistance phenomena. It is for this reason and being a parasite of potential zoonotic risk that at present pharmacological tests have been developed in the search for new alternatives for the treatment of giardiasis, especially in the canine and feline species as mentioned earlier.

Keywords: benzimidazoles, *Giardia intestinalis*, imidazoles, nitazoxanide, teclozan

1. Introduction

Giardiasis is a parasitic disease, caused by a protozoan called *Giardia duodenalis*, which shares similar morphological characteristics with other species such as *G. lamblia* and *G. intestinal*, for which the same pathogen has been considered [1–3]; this protozoan affects many domestic and wild species [2]. In the canine and feline species, it is described as *G. intestinalis* [1, 2], previously described as *Giardia canis*; this protozoan affects not only animals but also man [4].

Epidemiology has been considered a cosmopolitan parasite, which causes malabsorption syndrome in the host, causing gastroenteritis in these patients [1, 4], due to the presence of giardia in intestinal mucosa, producing ulcerative lesions and hemorrhagic, it should be made clear that, not being an agent considered cosmopolitan, it does not affect the species of cattle such as cattle, goats, sheep, and swine [1, 2, 4], it is a seriously pathogenic agent for animal species, that if it causes injuries that produce a consuming disease, considered as a zoonotic disease of global importance [2].

The prevalence is higher in areas with unhealthy conditions [3, 5], where the presence of excreta in the water, excreta management, overcrowding, and warm conditions has been described, favoring the presence of an agent [6]. Transmission is oro-fecal; humans, canines, and felines ingest the infecting cysts [2, 3], which hatch and develop into gastroenteritis later on. This route allows the outbreaks between dogs and humans frequently, especially in rural areas and shelter canines [7, 8].

It is important to introduce ourselves in the treatment, to comment on the typical clinical signs of the disease, these are due to gastroenteritis [2], due to damage of the villi of the intestine, leading to malabsorption syndrome [8–10], this type of gastroenteritis causes not only typical diarrhea with mucus, odor, and steatorrhea, but also abdominal discomfort, vomiting, nausea, regurgitation, and anorexia. This is why it is important to use drugs that are not only extremely effective (greater than 95% effectiveness) but also the least gastrolesive or irritant.

For the treatment of giardiasis, there are a number of drugs approved by the Food and Drug Administration (FDA), which are described in the Plumb and Papich therapeutic manuals [11, 12]. It is important that it is established which drugs have kinetic studies in animal species, because sometimes pharmacological products are used, which has few studies in domestic species and if we speak of a health picture, not only high morbidity but zoonotic, it should be clear that products can be formulated and what are their therapeutic indications, according to previous studies.

The drugs used for the curative treatment of *G. intestinalis* will be categorized into pharmacological groups, which will indicate their most relevant pharmacological characteristics, such as the mechanism by which the agent is eliminated, its kinetic behavior, contraindications to be taken into account when given, and the dose suggested by the effectiveness studies.

The prevalence of *G. intestinalis* in canines of Colombia is unknown, since the studies described for the canine species are pitifully isolated, whereas in other parts of world, it has been estimated that the prevalence is at 7% and for South America, the prevalence is 27.6%. In Colombia, Alarcón et al. (2015) reported a prevalence of 0.81% in a study with 122 samples of fecal matter in Bogotá, whereas Caraballo et al. (2007) in the center of veterinary medicine and zootechnics CES, Envigado, Colombia, reported a prevalence of 13.9%, compared with research in 22 canine refuges that Sierra-Cifuentes et al. (2015) conducted and a prevalence of 6.8 and 10.3% for the municipality of Medellín and Oriente Antioqueño, respectively.

2. Therapeutic of giardiasis

2.1. Nitroimidazole

This group of drugs is the most described for the treatment of giardiasis, in many countries of the world, both for dogs and for cats, and is one of the most described pharmacological products in the treatment of giardiasis in humans [13–15].

Nitroimidazole class drugs, which are considered to be anti-Giardia, have some limitations in domestic species, especially in small animals, where their toxic effects on the central nervous system (CNS) have been described when close doses have been used at 50 mg/kg [16], especially in felines; other authors suggest not exceeding the dose of 25 mg/kg in felines [11].

Within the nitroimidazole family of drugs, metronidazole, secnidazole, tinidazole, and dimetridazole are frequently used in the treatment of intestinal protozoa, such as *Entamoeba histolytica, Trichomona fetus,* and *G. intestinalis,* in some animal species and in man [17–19]. As for the treatments of giardiasis, we will try to elucidate which are the most updated therapies for the treatment of these parasites. To understand this group of drugs and as their routine use is important to understand the mechanism of action, nitroimidazoles have antibacterial and antiprotozoal mechanism of action and generate nitrogen radicals, which affect the metabolism of the parasite or bacteria. These drugs disrupt the DNA of organisms through a reaction with intracellular metabolites [11, 12, 17].

With regard to their pharmacological characteristics, the oral absorption of nitroimidazoles is almost complete by the oral route, but are somewhat gastrolesivos, especially in humans which cause anorexia and give a metallic taste to the mouth [20]; in horses, their bioavailability is of 75–100%, whereas in felines and canines, it is 60–100% [12] in dogs. This group of drugs has variable mean lives according to the species: 2–4 h in horses, 9–12 h in foals, 4–5 h in dogs, and 4.8 h in cats [12, 17, 21], given mainly in urine [18]. In cats, metronidazole benzoate salt has been used or suggested, which improves palatability.

As for the adverse effects of these drugs, CNS toxicity is described mainly by several authors; as mentioned previously, doses close to 50 mg/kg cause especially in feline states of lethargy, depression, ataxia, incoordination, tremors, vomiting, weakness, and clonic seizures. The explanation of this phenomenon of drug toxicity is mainly due to the fact that nitroimidazoles cause an inhibition of gamma butyric acid (GABA). Peripheral neuropathic lesions can also be frequent in doses higher than 25 mg/kg [11, 12, 16].

Due to their hepatic metabolism that is achieved by the action of cytochrome P450, by hydroxylation, and conjugation with glucuronic acid, they can cause toxic liver diseases after continuous use [18]. It is important to emphasize that by their oral presentation, these drugs have the property of causing states of inappetence, especially in dogs and cats [17, 18], so their use has been lost for the treatment of giardiasis in these species, because the agent of per se causes inappetence which can be potentiated, after the use of these drugs.

It is important to document that these drugs are mutagenic and teratogenic and therefore should not be used in pregnant females. It is also important to note that the addition of salts to improve the taste can also cause harmful effects especially in cats that are intolerant to acid derivatives, benzoic acid [12].

Regarding therapeutics, it has been described that metronidazole is 100% effective for the treatment of giardia enteritis; the explanation is based not only on its ability to eliminate other common agents such as amoebas and trichomonas, which may be parasitizing concomitantly, but also on its property of inhibiting the lymphocytic response behaving as an intestinal anti-inflammatory at the same time [16, 17].

The recommended dose for domestic species varies according to the drug, species and agent to be treated, as for metronidazole, 22 mg/kg every 12 h for 5 days [11, 21]; for canines, Papich suggests not exceeding 15 mg/kg every 12 h for 8 days; and in cats, it is suggested 10–25 mg/kg every 12 h for 8 days [11, 12, 21, 22]. Other authors recommend an effective dose of 100% for cats of 22–25 mg/kg every 12 h for 5–7 days [16, 23]. For the author, 20 mg/kg has been shown to be an effective dose for canines and felines every 12 h for 5 days [17].

Other nitroimidazoles such as tinidazole 44 mg/kg every 24 h for 3 days have also been used in small animals [21]; while Papich only indicates that 15 mg/kg every 12 h for 5 days is sufficient for dogs and cats [22], secnidazole 30 mg/kg single dose is recommended in a study conducted in a canine shelter and found effectiveness of 725 with a single dose [24].

Other nitroimidazoles, such as ipronidazole, ornidazole, and ronidazole, which have been used in the treatment of giardiasis in a small number of animals, some medicated in drinking water, have been suggested for use in birds than for canines and felines [17–19].

2.2. Benzimidazoles

The benzimidazoles are a group of drugs that have frequently been used for the treatment of parasitic nematodes mainly, although their effectiveness in the control of cestodes and trematodes has been evident. Its capacity to eliminate not only the adult forms but also the ovoposición has been the treatment of gastrointestinal parasites in many animal species [17–19], including humans, where this group is of greater importance in the control of giardias [13, 15].

Nowadays, benzimidazoles and especially fenbendazole and its prodrug febantel are considered as the standard drugs for the control of canine and feline giardiasis [25], not only because of its effectiveness, which is 100% [26, 27], but also because they require fewer days of treatment as well as a longer half-life, which facilitates their administration especially in small animals.

Within this group of drugs, there are two that have been shown to be effective for the treatment of *G. intestinalis*, which are fenbendazole and albendazole, the latter widely used in humans for the treatment of giardiasis in children [13, 15, 28].

It is important to document some of the pharmacodynamic properties of the benzimidazoles. Its mechanism of action is to produce the degeneration of the parasite microtubule and irreversibly block the uptake of glucose by the parasite; in this case, *Giardia* spp. inhibit the uptake of glucose causing the depletion of energy reserves in the parasite and eventually resulting in death (Papich). However, there is no effect on host glucose metabolism, in this case mammal, as indicated benzimidazoles have been used for the treatment of giardiasis in many animal species, not only dogs and cats, but also sheep, goats, and calves, which can also be parasitized by this zoonotic agent [11, 12, 22].

Regarding their kinetic behavior, benzimidazoles are absorbed marginally after oral administration; blood levels in calves are 0.11 μg/ml and in horses are 0.07 μg/ml, whereas in canines and felines at levels of up to 0.2 μg/ml, allowing it to have a high volume of distribution [11, 21], reaching sites where the parasites are in a hypobiotic form, hence showing their great quality in eliminating larvae in the state of hypobiosis. This family of drugs has a hepatic metabolism, by the simple action of the cytochromes P450, being the excretion between 44–50% by feces and 1% by urine.

It is important to describe that febantel is a prodrug, which presents first-pass metabolism, which transforms it after the metabolism in fenbendazole and albendazole, which makes it a very potent anti-giardia, by sum synergism [11, 17].

With regard to the safety of the drugs in this family, it is important to note that they are very safe, with a high safety margin, but they may also have some digestive problems such as vomiting and diarrhea, especially when doses higher than those suggested are given or intervals increased, such as three to five times a day [11, 12, 22]. In terms of renal and hepatic safety, the author has found that benzimidazoles are very safe for both kidney and liver and are also very safe during gestation and lactation; no known contraindications for domestic species have been described and used at any age [11, 17, 22].

Benzimidazole treatment for the management of *G. intestinalis* is based on three pharmacological products: fenbendazole, albendazole, and febantel; the treatment is with fenbendazole [26] or febantel [29], but due to constant reinfection and resistance phenomena, these have lost effectiveness. Goniostasis in canines can be treated with fenbendazole at a dose of 50 mg/kg as described by Barr et al. (1994); Zajac et al. (1998) [1], which has now been considered the treatment standard because it has a 100% effectiveness. This description is similar to those given by other authors but in species such as sheep (*Ovis orientalis*), where at a dose of 10 mg/kg once daily for three days is equally effective that in canines [30]; some authors, in particular Geurden et al., suggest that the standard dose in sheep for *G. intestinalis* should be 15 mg/kg every 24 h for 3 days [31]. In *Bos taurus* calves, the dose of fenbendazole is much smaller, where 5 mg/kg every 24 h oral for 3 days is effective in 90% [32].

In a study conducted by Molina, Salazar and Cabreraet (2016), it was found that fenbendazole was 60% effective for the control of *G. intestinalis* cysts and trophozoites at a dose of 50 mg/kg orally every 24 h for 3 days, which is similar to the descriptions made by other authors [30, 33, 34], but discusses the 100% effectiveness that documents for drug authors such as Montoya (2008), Villanueva (2009), and Meltzer, et al (2014) [26, 29, 35].

In cats, the treatment has been found to be effective with febantel 37.8 mg/kg, oral every 24 h for 5 days [23], whereas the dose in canines is equal, 100% effectiveness is achieved with only 3 days of treatment, in which the number of cysts in the proportion discussed above is eliminated [34].

The uses of other benzimidazoles such as albendazole at a dose of 25 mg/kg every 12 h for 4 days have been shown to be effective in killing infected animals [22]. However, therapy with albendazole may cause bone marrow suppression and therefore should be used with caution in canines and felines, in a case of acute giardiasis [22]. In sheep, the use of albendazole at doses of 20 mg/kg oral once daily is sufficient to control *G. intestinalis* [30], a situation very similar in humans.

Other benzimidazoles, such as mebendazole, have been found to be only 37% effective against giardiasis; thus their use is impractical [12].

2.3. Nitrofurans

Some authors have described the use of antibiotics for the treatment of *G. intestinalis*, especially in human therapy, in which the use of furazolidone has been routine for decades; in animal species, some authors such as Papich [22] and Plumb [11] indicate that this antibiotic has effectiveness against the parasite.

The study of the pharmacodynamics of this antibiotic will allow us to understand its giardicidal ability; furazolidone interferes with susceptible bacterial or parasitic enzymatic systems, within which we can indicate that it has activity against *Vibrio cholerae*, *Trichomonas fetus*, *Eimeria* spp., *Isospora* spp., *Neospora* spp., and many strains of *E. coli*, Enterobacter, Campylobacter, Salmonella, and Shigella. This antibiotic also has the property of inhibiting monoamine oxidase [11, 12, 22].

As for pharmacokinetics, the information is somewhat contradictory regarding the absorption characteristics of furazolidone; it is absorbed orally and reaches in the different body fluids, with concentrations sufficient to exert an effective antibacterial action. Its absorption is fast in the small intestine, but prefers media with acid pH, with little water solubility. Its metabolism is hepatic with a half-life of 30 min, and its binding to plasma proteins is 60%, which causes most of it to be excreted in urine [17–19].

The suggested dose for the treatment of giardiasis in dogs and cats is 4 mg/kg, orally every 12 h for 7 days [12, 22]; in the case of cats, it has been recommended that the dose should be given per 10 days [11, 21].

2.4. Quinacrine

This drug is currently one of the least used, basically because of its side effects that are sometimes annoying; this drug has properties and activities against a variety of protozoa and helminths. Its use against all except Giardia and Trichomonas has been replaced by agents safer or more effective [12, 21, 22], as we have already discussed.

In humans, quinacrine may be used for the treatment of mild-to-moderate discoid lupus erythromatosis (LE), transcervically as a sterilizing agent, or as a powder as an intrapleural sclerosing agent [11].

As for its mechanism of action, quinacrine has its antiprotozoal activity against Giardia not understood; however, it binds to DNA by intercalation at adjacent base pairs, thus inhibiting RNA transcription and translocation [11, 21, 22]. In addition, quinacrine interferes with electron transport and inhibits the oxidation of succinate and cholinesterase, which binds to nucleoproteins that (in humans at least) can suppress the lupus erythromatosis cell factor [11, 21].

To know its pharmacokinetics, this product is absorbed well from the gastrointestinal tract, after the oral administration. It is distributed throughout the body, but CSF levels are only 1–5% of those found in plasma [12, 22]. The drug is concentrated in the liver, spleen, lungs, and adrenals [21]. It is relatively highly limited to plasma proteins in humans (80–90%). This can pass through the placenta, but only small amounts enter the breast milk. The elimination is slow, with a half-life of 5 days, with a slow liver metabolism, being eliminated almost entirely by the kidney, causing acidification of the urine, which increases its excretion via this pathway [11, 21].

It is important to know that is contraindicated its use in behavioral alterations, psoriasis and porphyria, very described in humans, more studies are missing in animals; it is clear that it should be handled with care in patients with hepatic disorders, since jaundice appears in addition to digestive signs such as anorexia, nausea, vomiting, and diarrhea, abnormal behaviors ("biting with fly," agitation), pruritus, and fever. In addition to hypersensitivity, liver disease, anemia, corneal edema, and retinopathy, it should not be used in pregnant females to cross the placental barrier and also has milk elimination. In humans, it is responsible for hydrocephalus, and in rats, the neonatal mortality rate is increased. According to the FDA, this drug is category C, so it should not be used during gestation [11, 22].

While its therapeutic safety is poor, an overdose can cause death; the signs of intoxication are neurological, giving convulsions, delirium, and excitement, in addition to what was described above with gastrointestinal symptoms.

The recommended dosage for canines is 6.6 mg/kg every 12 h for 5 days [36]; other authors recommend 9 mg/kg orally every 24 h for 6 days [21]. For cats, the dose is 9 mg/kg, oral every 24 h for 6 days [37].

2.5. Paromomycin

It is an antibiotic of the aminoglycoside family, whose bactericidal effect is the irreversible inhibition of the 30 S subunit of bacterial chromosomes, preventing the formation of the initiation complex between mRNA and ribosome [17, 18, 38], thereby inhibiting protein synthesis.

This drug is considered as an amebicide and anthelmintic directly by contact, although its mechanism of action is unknown. In human medicine, it has been used for the treatment of mixed enteritis including giardiasis [13, 28]; in addition, it acts as an intestinal bactericide of digestive bacterial flora, including ammonia-producing bacteria [13, 15].

Paromomycin exhibits a broad spectrum of action, including bacteria, protozoa, and helminths. It is active mainly against amoebas such as *E. histolytica*. It also exhibits activity against Gram-negative bacteria and some Gram-positive bacteria such as Staphylococcus strains. It has some activity against *Mycobacterium tuberculosis*, but is totally ineffective in the case of *Pseudomonas aeruginosa*. Finally, it is anthelmintic in case of infections caused by *Diphyllobothrium latum*, *Dipylidium caninum*, *Hymenolepis nana*, *Taenia saginata*, and *Taenia solium* [15].

Regarding pharmacokinetics, after oral administration, absorption may increase in situations in which the permeability of the intestinal mucosa is altered, such as inflammation or erosion of the epithelium [13], and elimination is by feces and via the kidneys slowly [15].

The recommended dosage for canines is 125–160 mg/kg, every 12 h for 5 days [25].

2.6. Nitazoxanide

Nitazoxanide is a synthetic derivative drug of salicylamide, used as a broad-spectrum antiparasitic agent with proven effectiveness in protozoal infections and worms [9, 39–41]. It is approved for infections by parasites such as *G. lamblia* and Asacarididos in human patients [13, 15]; it is considered an extremely safe pediatric drug [28].

This drug, initially explored in the equine species, was indicated in horses for the treatment of equine protozoal myeloencephalitis (EPM) caused by *Sarcocystis neurone* [11, 21, 22]. In recent years, it has been explored in the canine species for the treatment of *G. intestinalis* [42].

The mechanism of action is to inhibit the enzyme pyruvate ferredoxin oxidoreductase (PFOR), disrupting the metabolism of the parasite; in addition, this mechanism prevents the transference of electrons preventing energy metabolism by the parasite [17]. In helminths, it inhibits the polymerization of tubulin in the parasite.

As far as pharmacokinetic data are concerned, they are well known in equines, where after oral administration, it is absorbed and transformed into tizoxanide (deacetyl-nitazoxanide); the maximum level is reached at 2–3 h; in humans, it is reached at 4 h, 99% of which is bound to plasma proteins [39], excreted by urine and bile, in the form of glucuronic acid [11, 22].

This drug is a prodrug, followed by its rapidly hydrolyzed administration to its active metabolite, tizoxanide, 99% of which binds to blood plasma proteins [39]. Peak concentrations are observed for 1–4 h after administration. It is excreted in the urine, bile, and feces [12]. Its mechanism of action is by the inhibition of tubulin in helminths [11]. In the case of protozoa, electron and biochemical resonance studies have shown that pyruvate ferridoxin oxidoreductase (PFOR) and, to a lesser extent, hydrogenase reduce ferredoxin, which is oxidized by the nitro group in position 5 over the nitroheterocyclic compounds such as nitazoxanide [39]. In these organisms, nitazoxanide is reduced to a toxic radical in an organelle of carbohydrate metabolism and the hydrogenosome which contains hydrogenase PFOR and ferredoxin [13, 15, 43].

After oral administration in horses, nitazoxanide is absorbed and rapidly converted to tizoxanide (deacetyl-nitazoxanide). Nitazoxanide levels are reached within 2–3 h and are not detectable 24 h after dosing, which is 99% bound to proteins and is metabolized in the liver and is excreted in urine, bile, and feces; glucuronic acid is the conjugation of the compound [39, 44].

Adverse effects are commonly reported, such as fever, anorexia, reduced appetite, lethargy, and depression (Rodríguez García et al., 2004, Delgado et al.). However, the reproductive safety of nitazoxanide has not been determined in pregnant females; it is categorized as drug B by the FDA, not used during gestation or lactation, and it has been considered that the LD 50 is 10 g/kg [11, 22, 39].

The recommended dosage for canines is 10 mg/kg every 24 h for 3 days [26]; in a study published by Cabrera and Molina, effectiveness found at 8 days of treatment was 43.75%, which increased at 30 days of treatment with 87.5% [45]. This finding differs from those found by other authors such as Moron-Soto et al. and other authors consulted [42, 46, 47], and totally contradictory with respect to human pediatric patients, where the effectiveness is 80% [48, 49].

2.7. Teclozan

In humans, one of the drugs of choice for protozoal infections is teclozan, which is a derivative of dichloroacetamide; its trade name is known as Falmonox® (Sanofi-Aventis®, Paris, France) and its dose varies between 25 and 50 mg/kg, every 24 h, for 5 days [17]. It is a drug of high efficacy and is considered safe, since it does not present teratogenic effects and its few side effects include flatulence, nausea, meteorism, headache, rush cutaneous, and urticaria. This drug acts in the intestinal lumen being effective in treating *G. intestinalis* [28].

The mechanism of action of teclozan in humans has been described as intervening in the phospholipid metabolism preventing the formation of arachidonic acid in the parasite, which has a lethal protozoan effect and has not been determined in studies in animal species [15, 17]. This product shows an efficiency of 60% in the treatment of giardiasis in children, when oral 10 mg/kg is given every 24 h [50]. It is important to discuss that the treatment of intestinal infections caused by protozoa and treated with teclozan has shown cure rates between 80 and 93% and with very few side effects and minimal relapse.

3. Other controls for giardiasis

There are vaccines for the control of Giardiasis of Fort Dodge© Animal Health for giardia, called Giardia-Vax® for dogs and Giardia Fel-O® for cats, their effectiveness being questionable [2, 51]. It has been considered that their application according to the commercial house, should be done after 4 months of life, and repetitions every 4–6 months, which makes its use in third world countries, is not very useful, if we consider epidemiological data on the prevalence of parasites in America Latin American countries, which can reach 27%, with high prevalences such as those in Brazil and Argentina that are above 20% (prevalence). This is why the use of the Giardia-Vax® vaccine in Latin America has had little impact on the control of the disease.

In human medicine, a combination of nutritional intervention and phytotherapy is the first line of approach for the treatment of giardiasis, whereas in veterinary medicine, dietary manipulation is often combined with antiprotozoal chemotherapy. Another point to consider is the use of probiotic therapy which could be useful in preventing infection or as an adjunct to the treatment of it; in this vein, the use of commensal bacteria can determine the vulnerability and the resistance to Giardia infection in mice. The use of probiotic lactobacilli releases a low molecular weight thermosensitive factor that inhibits the proliferation of Giardia trophozoites in in vitro culture. These modern therapeutic strategies justify further investigation which could prove to be more applicable and useful than drugs for the treatment in endemic regions [8, 52].

In any case, part of the control of the agent is to improve sanitary conditions, avoid contamination of water and food with cysts of the parasite, and control of more frequent parasites in hostile environments, that is, deworming programs every 3–4 months, especially for the canine species, with effective products such as benzimidazoles and especially fenbendazole and in particular the hygiene of pets with the use of baths with detergent products based on chlorhexidine, irgasan, and benzoyl peroxide (**Table 1**).

Drug	Dose canine	Dose feline
Metronidazole	10–25 mg/kg BID for 5–8 days	15–25 mg/kg BID for 8 days
Secnidazole	30 mg/kg SID for 1–3 days	
Tinidazole	10–44 mg/kg SID for 3 days	15 mg/kg BID for 3 days
Albendazole	25 mg/kg BID for 4 days	25 mg/kg BID for 4 days
Fenbendazole	50 mg/kg SID for 3 days	50 mg/kg SID for 3 days
Febantel	37.8 mg/kg SID for 3 days	37.8 mg/kg SID for 3 days
Furazolidona	4 mg/kg BID for 7 days	4 mg/kg BID for 7 days
Quinacrina	6.6–9 mg/kg SID, BID for 5–6 days	9 mg/kg BID for 6 days
Paromomicina	125–160 mg/kg BID for 5 days	
Nitazoxanida	10 mg/kg SID for 3 days	
Teclozan	10 mg/kg SID for 3 days	

Table 1. Drugs used in canines and felines for the treatment of giardia intestinalis.

Author details

Víctor Manuel Molina Díaz

Address all correspondence to: dooncanmc@hotmail.com

Corporación Universitaria Lasallista, Caldas, Colombia

References

[1] Bowman D. Protozoans. Georgis' parasitology for veterinarians. 8th ed. Saunders, editor. St Louis; 2009. p. 84-114

[2] Payne PA, Artzer M. The Biology and Control of *Giardia* spp and Tritrichomonas foetus. Veterinary Clinics of North America - Small Animal Practice. Elsevier Ltd; 2009;**39**(6):993-1007

[3] Caccio S, Thompson R, McLauchlin J, Smith H. Unravel-ling Cryptosporidium and Giardia Epidemiology. Trends Parasitol. 2005;**21**:430-7

[4] Adam R. Biology of Giardia lamblia. Clin Microbiol Rev. 2001;**14**(3):447-475

[5] Smith H, Caccio S, Cook N. Cryptosporidium and Giardia as foodborne zoonoses. Vet Parasitol. 2007;**149**(1-2):29-40

[6] Peralta ML, Ayala J. Algunas consideraciones sobre la prevalencia actual de entamoeba histolytica, *Giardia duodenalis*, coccidios, microsporidios y mixosporidios en Colombia. Salud Uninorte. 2008;**24**(2):294-302

[7] Meireles P, Montiani-Ferreira F, Thomaz-Soccol V. Survey of giardiasis in household and shelter dogs from metropolitan areas of Curitiba, Parana state, Southern Brazil: Vet Parasitol. 2008;**152**(34):242-8

[8] Thompson R. The zoonotic significance and molecular epidemiology of Giardia and giardiasis. Vet Parasitol. 2004;**126**:15-35

[9] Tejman-Yarden N, Millman M, Lauwaet T, Davids BJ, Gillin FD, Dunn L, et al. Impaired parasite attachment as fitness cost of metronidazole resistance in *Giardia lamblia*. Antimicrobial Agents and Chemotherapy. 2011;**55**(10):4643-4651

[10] Ringqvist E, Palm J, Skarin H. Release of metabolic enzymes by Giardia in response to interaction with intestinal epithelial cells. Molecular and Biochemical Parasitology. 2008;**159**(2):85-91

[11] Plumbs D. Veterinary Drugs Handbook. 7th ed. Publishing B, editor. Wisconsin; 2014. 1239 p.

[12] Riviere JE, Papich MG. Veterinary Pharmacology & Therapeutics. Novena. Iowa: Wiley-blackwell; 2009. 1525 p

[13] Brunton L, Lazo J, Parjer KL. Goodman & Gilman. The Pharmacological basis of therapeutics. Vol. Undécima. New York: McGraw Hill; 2007. 2045 p

[14] González-Mantilla JF. Farmacología, Terapeútica y Anestesiología en peces. In Bogotá; 2010. p. 50-62

[15] Dipiro JT, Talbert RL, Yee GC, Matzke GR, Well B, Posey M. Pharmacotherapy a pathophiologic approach. Vol. séptima. McGraw Hill; 2008

[16] Ettinger S, Feldman E. Tratado de Medicina Interna Veterinaria. Vol. sexta. Madrid: Elsevier; 2007

[17] Molina V. Farmacología veterinaria. 1st ed. Lasallista, editor. Medellín; 2016. 356 p

[18] Botana LM. Farmacología Veterinaria: Fundamentos y aplicaciones terapéuticas. 1st ed. Panamericana, editor. Buenos Aires; 2016. 482 p

[19] Sumano López H, Ocampo Camberos L. Farmacología veterinaria. Tercera. México: McGraw Hill; 2006. 1082 p

[20] González Carro MA. Vademécum de farmacología veterinaria en perros y gatos. México: Trillas; 2008. 172 p

[21] Plumb DC. Plumb´s Veterinary Drug Handbook. Seventh. Wiley-blackwell; 2011. 1594 p

[22] Papich MG. Saunders Handbook of Veterinary Grugs. Fourth. St Louis: Elsevier; 2016. 933 p

[23] Scorza AV, Ballweber LR, Tangtrongsup S, Panuska C, Lappin MR. Comparisons of mammalian *Giardia duodenalis* assemblages based on the β-giardin, glutamate dehydrogenase and triose phosphate isomerase genes. Veterinary parasitology [Internet]. 2012 Oct 26 [cited 2016 May 7];**189**(2-4):182-188. Available from: http://www.sciencedirect.com/science/article/pii/S0304401712002300

[24] Ramírez P, Ruiz JD, Múnera AM, Arroyave C, Castaño L, López P. Efectividad del secnidazol para el control de la Giardia spp. en caninos adultos [Internet]. Universidad CES; 2013. Available from: http://hdl.handle.net/10946/3171

[25] Greene CE. Infectious Diesease of the Dog and Cat. Fourth. St Louis: Elsevier; 2012. 1383 p

[26] Villeneuve A. Giardia y Cryptosporidium como agentes infecciosos emergentes. Veterinary focus. 2009;**19**(1):42-45

[27] Nelson RW, Couto G. Small Animal Internal Medicine. Fourth. St Louis: Mosby-Elsevier; 2009. 1499 p

[28] González MA, Lopera WD, Arango A. Fundamentos de Medicina: Manual de Terapéutica. Decima sex. Medellín: Corporación para Investigaciones Biologicas CIB; 2015. 758 p

[29] Montoya A, Dado D, Mateo M. Efficacy of Drontal(R) Flavour Plus (50 mg praziquantel, 144 mg pyrantel embonate, 150 mg febantel per tablet) against Giardia sp in naturally infected dogs. Parasitol Res. 2008;**103**(5):1141-1144

[30] Xiao L, Saeed K, Herd RP. Efficacy of albendazole and fenbendazole against Giardia infection in cattle. Veterinary Parasitology. 1996;**61**(1-2):165-170

[31] Geurden T, Pohle H, Sarre C, Dreesen L, Vercruysse J, Claerebout E. The efficacy of a treatment with fenbendazole against an experimental *Giardia duodenalis* infection in lambs. Small Ruminant Research. Elsevier B.V.; 2011;**96**(2-3):211-215

[32] O'Handley RM, Buret AG, McAllister TA, Jelinski M, Olson ME. Giardiasis in dairy calves: Effects of fenbendazole treatment on intestinal structure and function. International Journal for Parasitology. 2001;**31**(1):73-79

[33] Petri WA. Therapy of intestinal protozoa. Trends in Parasitology. 2003;**19**(11):523-526

[34] Payne A, Ridley K, Dryden W. Efficacy of a combination febantel-praziquantel-pyrantel product, with or without vaccination with a commercial Giardia vaccine, for treatment of dogs with naturally occurring giardiasis. J Am Vet Med A. 2002

[35] Meltzer E, Lachish T, Schwartz E. Treatment of giardiasis after nonresponse to nitroimidazole. Emerging Infectious Diseases. 2014;**20**(10):1742-1744

[36] Georgi J, Georgi M. Parasitología en clínica canina. México: Mc Graw-Hill Intermericana; 1994. 231 p

[37] Well B, editor. Adams, RH. (2001). Veterinary Pharmacology and Therapeutics (8a ed.). Iowa: Black well

[38] Botana L, Landoni F, Jiménez T. Farmacología y Terapéutica Veterinaria. 1st ed. Intermericana MG-H, editor. Madrid; 2002

[39] Zhao Z, Xue F, Zhang L, Zhang K, Fei C, Zheng W, et al. The pharmacokinetics of nitazoxanide active metabolite (tizoxanide) in goats and its protein binding ability in vitro. Journal of Veterinary Pharmacology and Therapeutics. 2010;**33**(2):147-153

[40] Belkind-Valdovinos U, Belkind-Gerson J, Sánchez-Francia D, Espinoza-Ruiz MM, Lazcano-Ponce E. Evaluación de la nitazoxanida en dosis única y por tres días en parasitosis intestinal. Salud Publica de Mexico. 2004;**46**(4):333-340

[41] Speich B, Ame SM, Ali SM, Alles R, Hattendorf J, Utzinger J, et al. Efficacy and safety of nitazoxanide, albendazole, and nitazoxanide-albendazole against trichuris trichiura infection: A randomized controlled trial. Plos Neglectd Tropical disease. 2012;**6**(6)

[42] Moron-soto M, Gutierrez L, Sumano H, Tapia G, Alcala-canto Y. Efficacy of nitazoxanide to treat natural Giardia infections in dogs. Parasites & Vectors; 2017;**10**(52):1-9

[43] Somvanshi VS, Ellis BL, Hu Y, Aroian RV. Nitazoxanide: Nematicidal mode of action and drug combination studies. Molecular and Biochemical Parasitology. Elsevier B.V.; 2014;**193**(1):1-8

[44] Goodman L, Gilman A, Hardman J, Limbird LE. Goodman & Gilman´s The Pharmacological basis of therapeutics. 12th ed. New York: McGraw Hill; 2006

[45] Cabrera A, Molina VM. De Un Albergue De Caldas , Antioquia , Colombia. Rev Cientifica FCV-LUZ. 2016;**XXVI**(6):389-396

[46] Hemphill A, Mueller J, Esposito M. Nitazoxanide, a broad-spectrum thiazolide anti-infective agent for the treatment of gastrointestinal infections. Expert Opin Pharmacother. 2006;**7**:953-964

[47] Soria-Arteche O, Hernández-Campos A, Yépez-Mulia L, Trejo-Soto PJ, Hernández-Luis F, Gres-Molina J, et al. Synthesis and antiprotozoal activity of nitazoxanide-N-methylbenzimidazole hybrids. Bioorganic and Medicinal Chemistry Letters. Elsevier Ltd; 2013;**23**(24): 6838-6841

[48] Gilles HM, Hoffman PS. Treatment of intestinal parasitic infections: A review of nitazoxanide. Trends in Parasitology. 2002;**18**(3):95-97

[49] Hoffman P, Sisson G, Croxen M. Antiparasitic drug nitazoxanide inhibits the pyruvate oxidoreductases of Helicobacter pylori, selected anaerobic bacteria and parasites, and Campylobacter jejuni. Antimicrob. Agents Chemother. Vol. Antimicrob Agents Chemother. 2007;**51**(3):868-876

[50] Mendieta-Chispe P, Avila-Stagg D. Entamoeba histolytica durante el embarazo: patogenia y tratamiento. Rev Med. 2000;**6**(4):260-262

[51] Castro-Hermida JA, González-Warleta M, Mezo M. Cryptosporidium spp. and *Giardia duodenalis* as pathogenic contaminants of water in Galicia, Spain: the need for safe drinking water. International journal of hygiene and environmental health [Internet]. 2015 Jan [cited 2016 May 7];**218**(1):132-138. Available from: http://www.sciencedirect.com/science/article/pii/S1438463914000820

[52] Thompson RCA. Giardiasis: Conceptos modernos sobre su control y tratamiento. 2008;**6150**:23-29

Chapter 9

Risk Assessment for *Giardia* in Environmental Samples

Ana Paola Balderrama-Carmona,
Gortáres-Moroyoqui Pablo,
Morán-Palacio Edgar Felipe,
Ulloa-Mercado Ruth Gabriela,
Díaz-Tenorio Lourdes Mariana and
Leyva-Soto Luis Alonso

Additional information is available at the end of the chapter

http://dx.doi.org/10.5772/intechopen.70805

Abstract

Giardia is a gastrointestinal parasite that causes infections in humans worldwide. In developing countries, giardiasis is an emerging infection because it plays an important role in diarrhea outbreaks linked to water and food consumption affecting the population in general. Giardiasis is referred to as zoonosis because its biological etiological agent is transmitted to humans through animal reservoirs by oral-fecal route. Detection and occurrences of *Giardia* cysts have been documented in water, food, soil, and air. The principal risk factors for developing giardiasis include environmental contamination associated with malnutrition and immunosuppression. The small size of cysts and their environmental resistance together with the small infection dose to produce the disease allow giardia dissemination especially in marginalized populations; however, parasitism is present in all countries and at different economic levels. This zoonotic illness contains several species of *Giardia duodenalis*, infecting mammals and humans with eight serotypes, of which A and B are of public health importance. Quantitative microbiological risk assessment (QMRA) is a methodology used for predicting health risk to establish regulations for permissible *Giardia* risk in water and food. This chapter focuses on worldwide reviews of *Giardia* incidence in environmental samples including giardiasis prevalence, serotypes, risk factors, and finally options for cyst reduction in the environment, emphasizing on QMRA.

Keywords: water, air, soil, food, giardiasis

1. Introduction

Gastrointestinal diseases have caused up to 871,000 deaths worldwide, which have been related to unsafe drinking water, health, and hygiene. Mortality rate is greater in African countries where death risk is 4.3×10^{-1} [1, 2]. Such data justify that the main risk factors are unsafe water and deficient cleaning linked to malnutrition and immunosuppression, invariable characteristics in marginalized communities. The microscopic parasite *Giardia* is among the main pathogens that cause gastrointestinal diseases at world level. In developing countries, 200 million people have been diagnosed with giardiasis symptoms, which are related to inadequate sanitation problems and access to safe drinking water. Giardiasis does not make a distinction between humans and animals by fecal-oral transmission using different routes: zoonotic, anthropogenic environmental, food, and water [3–5].

The strategy used in this research was assessed by analyzing different literature studies related to *Giardia* risk assessment; the search was performed in databases from October 2000 to October 2016, using the following terms: giardiasis risk factors; *Giardia* cysts in water, air, soil, and food; quantitative microbial risk assessment (QMRA); and cyst treatments. No restriction was found in language. This chapter focuses on reviewing world incidence of *Giardia* in water, soil, air, and food, including giardiasis prevalence, risk factors, and finally a system to reduce cysts in the environment, emphasizing on QMRA.

2. *Giardia* generalities

Giardia is one of the most primitive eukaryotic protozoa initially described by Leeuwenhoek in 1681; its taxonomy was confusing and complicated throughout the first half of the twentieth century. The name *Giardia lamblia* was well-known in the 1970s, but it was consolidated and changed to *Giardia duodenalis* or *Giardia intestinalis* in the 1990s. It is classified within the class Zoomastigophorea in the order Diplomaida and family Hexamitidae. Historically, 41 species have been described based on their hosts. To date, eight of these species have been detected in mammals: *duodenalis, enterica, canis, bovis, muris, cati, simondi,* and *microti* (**Table 1**) [6–9].

Giardia exists in two forms: an active form called a trophozoite and an inactive form called a cyst. The cyst measures 5 × 7 to 10 μm in diameter, containing four nuclei covered by a wall from

Species*	Host
G. intestinalis	Humans and mammals
G. agilis	Amphibian
G. muris	Rodents
G. ardeae	Birds
G. psittaci	Birds
G. microti	Rats and moles

Table 1. Giardia species.

0.3 to 0.5 μm in thickness; it is composed of an exterior filament layer formed by glycoproteins and an internal membrane layer that makes it very resistant providing an environmentally stable life cycle; it helps withstanding long periods in water at temperatures less than 25°C, and it even makes it invulnerable to chlorination processes. Trophozoites are pear-shaped and are approximately 12–15 mm in length and 5–9 mm in width with a cytoskeleton that includes a medium size body, four pairs of flagella, and a ventral disk; they have two nuclei without nucleoli in its interior, which are found in front and symmetrically located [10, 11].

The vital cycle of *Giardia* starts with the ingestion of cysts by the host whether found in food or water contaminated with feces of the infection carriers; once consumed, the cyst enters in contact with the gastric acid destroying itself and excystation occurs and trophozoites are released, which pass through the upper small intestine infecting the duodenum and the upper part of the intestine where they are reproduced by binary fission adhering to the intestinal epithelium surface and triggering symptomatology. The adaptation mechanism of *Giardia* known as encystment is essential to the parasite for their survival once out of the intestine of the host since trophozoites are extremely sensitive to changes in temperature, humidity, and the presence of chemical agents. In this process, trophozoites descend through the host intestine, and when they find a cholesterol-poor environment, their differentiation to cysts is induced and eliminated with feces. It has been reported that infected persons excrete from 10^8 to 10^9 cysts in only one evacuation and can continue discarding them from 50 days and including months later after diarrhea has subsided [10, 12].

For the parasite to survive within the host and avoid the immune response, *Giardia* shows what is known as antigenic variation that allows it to elude the immunologic system and produce chronic and recurrent infection. Giardiasis symptoms in human beings show variable degrees. Acute giardiasis shows acute diarrhea and urticaria or it can show itself asymptomatically; the acute form is usually self-limiting lasting for 2–7 days; it is also possible to evolve to a subacute or chronic stage lasting from months to years; malabsorption results as the most frequent and harmful complication difficult to solve from a therapeutic point of view because it causes malnutrition and low weight [13–15].

3. Giardiasis epidemiology

3.1. *Giardia* in the environment

The necessary dosage for giardiasis to start is from 10 cysts, which have been found in all environmental matrices: water, soil, air, and food. In drinking water, up to 24 cysts/L have been reported [16]; 87 cysts/L in soil; 0.0087 cysts/L in air [17]; and 40 cysts/L in leafy vegetables [18]. Most research has monitored *Giardia* cysts in water (**Table 2**). Giardiasis life cycle includes illness in several mammal species mediated by the environment, which is why climate factors such as humidity and temperature influence in cyst exposure, which are very persistent and their viability is preserved more in temperate and humid climates. *Giardia* cysts can maintain their infectious capacity from 15 days up to 2 months in water; 15 days to 1 month in soil; and from 2 to 10 days in vegetables; because of their small size and weight, they can be found suspended in air. Their resistance in the environment is a natural advantage to invade new hosts and expand their

Source	Location	Percent positive*	(oo)cyst 100 L^{-1}*	Reference
Waste water	EU, Italy, Ireland, Spain	25–100	3.2×10^3–4.2×10^4	[19–22]
Surface water	Belgium, Germany, Ireland, the Netherlands, Malaysia, Taiwan, EU, México, China	10–81	0.2–18.6 × 10^4	[23–27]
Drinking water	Bulgaria/Russia, Spain	5–27	0–62	[28, 29]
Ground water	Bulgaria/Russia, Brazil, France	8–62.5	6–3.61 × 10^3	[29–32]

Table 2. Occurrence and density of Giardia cyst in water.

progeny, which is why they have been identified as a potential danger to food products that are equally contaminated with animal feces or with contaminated water [17, 32]. Fecal runoff and vectors increase pathogen dissipation and thus the risk of acquiring the disease [33].

3.2. Genotypes

Giardia has many species characterized, but *G. intestinalis*, *lamblia*, or *duodenalis* is more recognized as a pathogen for human beings and a wide range of hosts including wild animal species. Currently, eight genetic groups from A to H (**Table 3**) are recognized; nonetheless, the species that are harmful for humans are divided into two genotypes: A (or Polish) and B (or Belgian), of which B is the most pathogenic in man [34]. Recent studies have revealed that genotype E has also been identified in humans [32].

The majority of research studies report that genotypes A and B have been found in clinical samples, and their distribution in the world is related to social and economic factors. The mix of both genetic groups (A and B) has also been reported in one sample, which suggests multiple infections [1] and confirms constant exposure to contaminated sources. It is common to find assemblages or genotypes A and E in superficial water [27].

Giardia genotypes can appear mixed as in the case of Scotland where both genotypes turn up, of which A is more prevalent [35]; the same case happened in Malaysia [36] and in Egypt, where A subtype I was the most prevalent [37]. In Latin America, particularly in Mexico, genotype A

Genotype	Hosts
A	Humans, cats, dogs, horses, calves, pigs, deers, lemurs, beavers, Guinea pigs, and sloths
B	Humans, dogs, monkeys, beavers, rabbits, guinea pigs, muskrats, and chinchilla
C, D	Dogs
E	Cows, goats, lams, and pigs
F	Cats
G	Rats
H	Marine vertebrates

Table 3. Recognized *Giardia* genotypes.

type II is only present [38]. While in Argentina, genotype A type II showed low seroprevalence, genotype B was found in high number of cases that included children and adults [39].

Genotype A is linked to diarrhea [40] and more in human origin than in zoonotic [1]; in disagreement, another study indicated that humans are the greatest source of assemblage B and that domestic animals are the greatest hosts of assemblage A [41].

3.3. Outbreaks and risk factors

An outbreak is a spontaneous increase of a disease occurrence. These cases are epidemiologically linked with at least one confirmed laboratory case. Numerous giardiasis outbreaks transmitted in water have occurred in the USA, Canada, England, France, Australia, Japan, and other industrialized nations due to contamination of water and food sources (**Table 4**). The factors that could be attributed to the increase of parasitic disease outbreaks produced by water and food are diverse. The increase of international travelers and migrants produces a rapid dissemination of the symptoms. Globalization of food sources, food imports as exotic fruits and vegetables are now necessary to satisfy consumption demands. Unfortunately, transportation conditions as controlled temperature have favored parasite survival in fruits and vegetables [50].

Two significant factors that contribute to the risk of contracting giardiasis are age and gender. Children from 1 to 5 years of age are more prone to the disease; in addition, infection incidence is greater in men than in women [38]. Divers have a high risk of contracting parasitosis even more than swimmers [51].

3.4. Impact in public health

Political, legal, economic, and public health is very committed to having reliable and safe drinking water sources for human consumption. An important concern is having them contaminated with pathogenic microorganisms such as *G. intestinalis*. The World Health Organization

Source	Location	Quantity of cases	Reference
Water sources	New Zealand	14	[42]
Swimming pool	Victoria, Australia	30	[43]
Drinking water	New Hampshire, EU	31	[44]
Water sources	New York, EU	36	[45]
Recreational water	California, EU	50	[46]
Water supply	Izmir; Turkey	196	[47]
Food/water	Scotland	185	[35]
Contaminated water	Bergen, Norwegian	2500	[48]
Foodborne/anthropogenic	All states in EU	19,140	[49]

Table 4. Giardiasis outbreaks.

(WHO) estimates that at least 10^9 cases of gastrointestinal diseases occur per year in one-third of the countries in the world, causing mortality of more than 5×10^6 persons at early age. The economic costs of diseases are alarming and cause financial losses. For this reason, social institutions have decided to work in developing better techniques for researching and controlling parasites in such a way that water turns out to be a safe liquid. Knowing the relative importance of specific transmission routes of intestinal protozoa, including potential sources of environmental contamination, constitutes fundamental aspects that allow understanding the epidemiology of parasitic diseases. In this manner, corrective measures can be applied to minimize prevalence and incidence of these diseases in the population. In developed countries, giardiasis is an emerging infection because it plays an important role in diarrhea outbreaks linked to water and food consumption that affect the population in general. As to developing countries in Asia, Africa, and Latin America, approximately 200 million people experience giardiasis symptoms [1, 52].

4. Detection methods in the environment

Detection techniques in environmental samples are diverse. Molecular biology methods are used to differentiate genotypes by using hybridization DNA probe DNA and polymerase chain reaction (PCR) techniques, starting from diverse fragments of nucleic acids as ribosomal RNA, los genes *hsp* 70, and random amplification of polymorphic DNA fragments (RAPD). The advantages of PCR techniques include high sensitivity, rapid analysis of several samples, relatively low cost, simultaneous detection of several pathogens, and the capacity to discriminate among several species of strains. These techniques are used mainly to differentiate *Giardia* species and genotypes [40].

The techniques to number *Giardia* cysts are those that use fluorescent antibodies; they can also differentiate viable and nonviable cysts by phase-contrast imaging [53]. Immunofluorescent microscopy techniques are used to detect *G. intestinalis* in water. The methods endorsed by the United States Environmental Protection Agency (USEPA) are the Information Collection Request (ICR) method protozoans (1999) and the 1623 method (2005). For water samples, this method is based on elution and purification of a filter stained with fluorescent monoclonal antibodies to then count the structures in a brilliant apple green color in an epifluorescence microscope (**Figure 1**). Many of these methods have already been adapted to recover cysts in food [54].

Fluorescent staining as acridine orange, propidium iodide (PI), and 4,6-diamidino-phenylindole (DAPI) are prone to have false positives and have variable stain characteristics depending on the viability state of the microorganism; nonetheless, the use of these stains, especially DAPI, can be very useful in identification when used together with other microscopy techniques such as fluorescence and phase contrast and differential interference contrast (DIC) [53].

Immunomagnetic separation (IMS) methods and the 1623 method have been developed to concentrate bacteria and protozoan pathogens. These methods use specific antibodies on the surface of paramagnetic particles to link target pathogens, followed by a magnet used to separate them

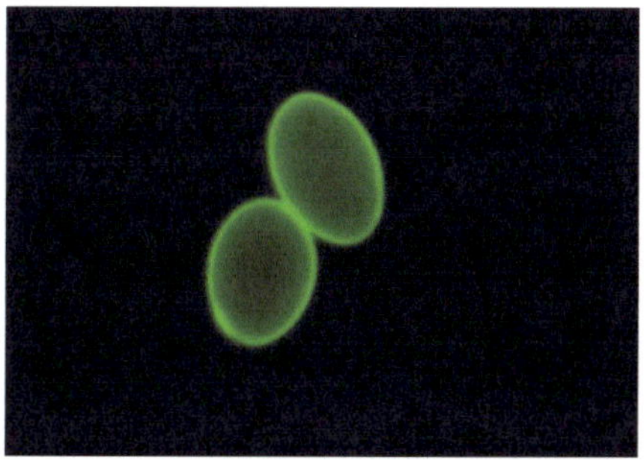

Figure 1. *Giardia intestinalis* cysts stained with fluorescent antibodies.

from the matrix sample [55]. The assay method of immunoabsorption linked to enzymes (ELISA) is more sensitive than the microscopy techniques for (oo)cyst detection [56].

Flux cytometry (FC) is a method by means of fluorescent activators capable of classifying cells according to their fluorescence and size. Detection and selective enumeration of *Giardia* cysts that are applied in FC consists of separating and observing the stained particles with immunofluorescent antibodies by the dispersion process. This method can potentially turn out to be the most precise in detecting and quantifying cysts [57].

Knowing cyst concentration in environmental samples and the necessary dosage when giardiasis starts allows us to estimate pathogen exposure; with this information and using the appropriate mathematic model, it is possible to calculate health risk. This methodology called quantitative microbial risk assessment (QMRA) is based on a series of steps that convey predicting daily and annual risks. In developed countries, QMRA has been adapted to assess permissible risk limits for *Giardia* in drinking water samples where the accepted risk worldwide is one infection for each 10,000 individuals.

5. Quantitative microbial risk assessment

The Codex Committee on Food Hygiene and the National Advisory Committee on Microbiological Criteria for Foods have proposed a framework for conducting QMRA. These guidelines also provide methods and approaches used to evaluate potential health effects and assess risks from contaminated source media, i.e., soil, air, and water. One of the key benefits of this method is the development of models describing the complex nature of pathogen populations in water or food supply [58].

Hazard identification involves pathogen detection in terms of concentration in water, for example. Next is exposure assessment where the quantity of water consumed for the people at risk is determined. In these two steps, one should take into account the recovery efficiency of the method, the characteristics of the people (age, sex, immune state, and customs), and pathogen survival. Then, the dose-response curve is calculated with the mathematical models described in the literature; finally, the integration of all the parameters provides the risk characterization that results in the likelihood of infection risk per day and year per person [59].

Quantitative microbial risk assessment has become a standard; the UK has pronounced a mandate that establishes that risk assessment be carried out by local government on many water supplies [60]. The US Environmental Protection Agency (EPA) handled permissible water *Giardia* risk values of <1:10,000 (10^{-4}) in a yearly exposure [61]. In the UK, the Water Supply Regulations 1999, and The New Dutch Drinking Water Decree state that for pathogenic microorganisms, health risk should be less than 1 infection/10,000 consumer/ year [62]. These risk regulations are equal to those of EPA. Developed countries are in the position to provide guidance, training, information resources, and technical assistance to advance supports for water safety. Thus, greater cooperation and collaboration at all levels should be effective and ensure that QMRA, as a water safety tool, will be available to all countries.

6. Quantitative microbial risk assessment for *Giardia* in environmental samples

The QMRA is an approach that has been widely used around the world to estimate the risk of infection by giardiasis in different sources of exposure. Most research studies have been performed in water samples, but the method has been applied in food, soil, and air samples.

In the last few years, the most relevant studies where QMRA has been used to evaluate giardiasis infection risks are the following:

In New Jersey, USA, the risk by accidental water ingestion (50 mL) of the Lower Passaic River was assessed resulting in a probability of 1:1 [23]. In Amsterdam, risk probability was calculated from 9×10^{-4} to 1.2×10^{-2} in recreational waters [63], while in Eastern Europe a giardiasis risk was predicted from 3×10^{-1} for water consumption from a well contaminated with sewage water [64]. In Mexico, a risk of 1.09×10^{-2} was estimated by lettuce consumption [65].

In France and England, *Giardia* risks were assessed due to water consumption from private well with values from 5.8×10^{-1} and 5.7×10^{-1}, respectively [60]. Risk for swimming in recreational waters of the Great Lakes in the USA was 5×10^{-3} [66]. The risk for rainwater consumption was also calculated in Australia at 3.1×10^{-1} [67].

In Brazil, giardiasis risk for drinking water consumption was estimated at 1.92×10^{-2} [68]. In Venezuela, the risk for bathers swimming in seawater was 3.6×10^{-2} [69]. In Switzerland, the risk by indirect contact with water from a lagoon contaminated with residual water was 3.5×10^{-1} [70], whereas risk by joint exposure to soil and dust transported by air was assessed at 1:1 in a rural town in Mexico [17].

In all the previous studies (**Figure 2**), the risks were greater than those allowed by the regulating commissions (1×10^{-4}), which is why these studies show that the microorganism concentration is enough to produce the disease in a percentage of the populations.

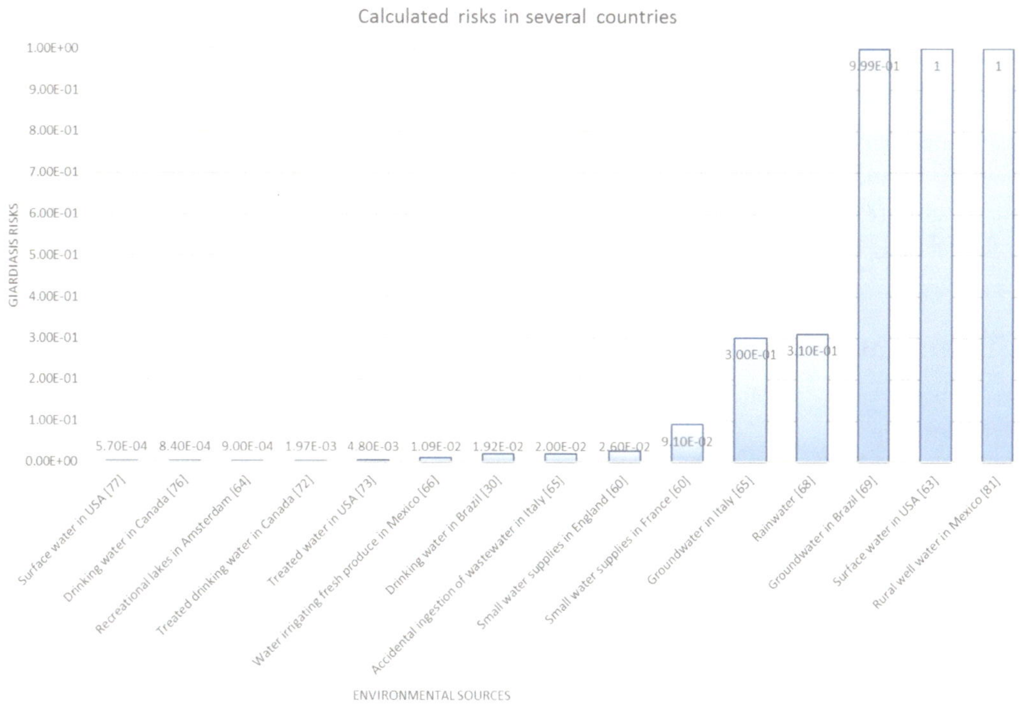

Figure 2. Risks by giardiasis calculated by quantitative microbial risk assessment in different countries.

Source	Location	Annual risk	Reference
Drinking water	Québec, Canada	8.4×10^{4}	[73]
Reclaimed water	California, EU	1.58×10^{-1}	[74]
Surface water	NJ, EU	1	[23]
Surface water	Arizona, EU	4.2×10^{-4}	[25]
Urban flooding	Netherlands	6×10^{-3}	[75]
Treated water	Saint Lawrence River, Canada	1.46×10^{-3}	[71], [73]
Tank water	Queensland, Australia	1.2×10^{-1}	[67]
Small water supplies	England	9.1×10^{-2}	[60]
	France	2.6×10^{-2}	
Well water	Sao Paulo, Brazil	9.9×10^{-1}	[30]
Drinking water	Zhejiang, China	6.25×10^{-6}	[76]
Drinking water	Sao Paulo, Brazil	1.92×10^{-2}	[69]
Tap water	Gorges Reservoir, China	1.3×10^{-1}	[27]
Reclaimed water	Tianjin, China	9.83×10^{-3}	[77]
Well water	Sonora, Mexico	9.9×10^{-1}	[17]
Small private systems	Canada	3.3×10^{-2}	[5]

Table 5. Annual risks of Giardia infections in different regions in the world.

Based on this information, it should be solved how to make these sources not harmful for humans and implement the necessary treatments for decreasing or eradicating giardiasis risk.

Using the concentrations reported in the literature, annual risk by giardiasis was calculated. To estimate infection probabilities (P_i), a consumption exposure of 1.46 L was taken into account [71], and then the exponential model equation $P_i = 1-\exp^{(-rN)}$ was used where $r = 0.0199$ [72] (**Table 5**).

7. Treatments decrease giardiasis risk

7.1. Water

It has been proven that the use of effective removal treatments for *Giardia* in water decreases the risk of acquiring the disease considerably. According to Surface Water Treatment Rule (SWTR), a series of requirements for superficial and underwater treatments were developed, which specify a removal or minimum inactivation of 3 log for *Giardia* [61].

The stabilization ponds are biological treatment systems that consist of excavated deposits with the sufficient surface and volume to provide the treatment periods; depending on oxygen requirements, the artificial lagoons can be aerobic, facultative, and anaerobic; it has been reported that these lagoons eliminate up to 2 logarithmic units of *Giardia* cysts. Stabilization ponds are the most conventional and it does not reach the minimum requirements for cyst removal according to the EPA; only does aerobic digestion reach 1.3 log of *Giardia* removal [11]; as to the water treatment with coagulation-flocculation only two logarithmic units of removal were achieved [78].

Currently, the best *Giardia* cyst removal treatments consist of using activated mud together with UV disinfection, with which 3.6 logarithmic units of cyst removal are reached [79]. The future bets on removing water contaminants by nanotechnological compounds, for example, nanocompounds of clay polymers and nanoadsorbents based on carbon and polymerics. Besides being effective, these compounds are economic [80].

7.2. Food

After water, the most important infection route with *Giardia* cysts is by food. The infections caused by these parasites are greatly the result of bad hygiene of the person responsible for food preparation. *Giardia* is always found coinfecting with other microorganisms, such as *Cryptosporidium, Vibrio cholerae,* and *Rotavirus* [81].

The consumption of raw food increases the risk of infection, which is why international recommendations exist to provide innocuousness in food preparation. It is especially important to (1) practice adequate hand hygiene for protection against this parasite; (2) buy food from reliable providers; (3) maintain food packed or closed; (4) perform pest control frequently; (5) make sure refrigerator temperature is below 5°C; (6) avoid cross-contamination by surfaces and recipients; (7) separate cooked from raw food; (8) use purified or boiled water especially if food is consumed raw; and (9) make sure food is cooked at high temperatures (≥70°C).

One of the main regulators of food innocuousness is the system ISO 22000, which is a combination of preliminary programs, such as the hazard analysis and critical control point (HACCP) principles, the implementation steps defined by the *Codex Alimentarius* Commission (CAC) and the regulated components of the norm ISO 9001:2000 [82].

8. Impact of climate change on giardiasis epidemiology

Climatic change is actually being considered as a triggering infection risk factor of zoonotic diseases because certain temperature conditions may increase the pathogens' infective capacity. In the case of *Giardia* cysts, the temperature may be a determining factor in its propagation because an increase in temperature may promote transmission although at low temperatures the cysts viability remains stable [33]; it may be due to increased intake of contaminated water either for drinking or using it for recreational activities [43].

Escobedo et al. [83] in their ecological study verified statistically that giardiasis increases significantly during the climate change that occurs with the "El Niño" phenomenon by using nonlinear Poisson models similar to those in QMRA and proving that *Giardia* infections are sensitive to climate. This knowledge can be helpful to identify sources of infection and support in the prevention and control of these diseases. Besides temperature, other factors that can increase the risk of giardiasis and directly related with climate change are precipitation/humidity and wind/dust [84].

9. Conclusions

Giardiasis outbreak studies have been reported worldwide with occurrence of *Giardia* cysts values up to still 100%; however, a continuous environmental examination is expensive, and it does not offer the necessary information about giardiasis reduction. QMRA is an approach indicated for determining risk infection probability due to pollution with cysts in water, food, soil, and air. It permits researching about the probable cause of pollution and the adequate treatment process. The high capacity of *Giardia* to infect (because of the large number of oocysts in the environment and the low dose necessary to infect) turns it into a serious world health risk. Therefore, it is important to create correct worldwide regulations designed for developing safety measurements of water, soil, air, and food sources.

Acknowledgements

The authors would like to thank Grelda Yañez and Diana Dorantes for editorial services in English.

Author details

Ana Paola Balderrama-Carmona[1], Gortáres-Moroyoqui Pablo[2], Morán-Palacio Edgar Felipe[1], Ulloa-Mercado Ruth Gabriela[2], Díaz-Tenorio Lourdes Mariana[2] and Leyva-Soto Luis Alonso[2]*

*Address all correspondence to: azospirillum_leyva@yahoo.com

1 Chemical-Biological and Agricultural Sciences Department, University of Sonora (UNISON) Southern Regional Unit, Navojoa, Sonora, México

2 Biotechnology and Food Sciences Department, Technological Institute of Sonora (ITSON), Cd. Obregon, Sonora, México

References

[1] Heredia RD, Hernández C, León C, Moncada L, Reyes P, Pinilla A, López M. Molecular diagnosis and genotype analysis of *Giardia duodenalis* in asymptomatic children from a rural area in central Colombia. Infection, Genetics and Evolution. 2015;**32**:208-213. DOI: 10.1016/j.meegid.2015.03.015

[2] World Health Organization. Monitoring Health for SDG. Switzerland: WHO Press; 2016. 136 p

[3] Durigan M, Abreu AG, Zucchi MI, Franco Regina MB, de Souza AP. Genetic diversity of *Giardia duodenalis*: Multilocus genotyping reveals zoonotic potential between clinical and environmental sources in a metropolitan region of Brazil. PLoS One. 2014;**9**(12):e115489. DOI: 10.1371/journal.pone.0115489

[4] Minetti C, Lamden K, Durband C, Cheesbrough J, Platt K, Charlett A, O'Brien SJ, Fox A, Wastling JM. Case-control study of risk factors for sporadic giardiasis and parasite assemblages in North West England. Journal of Clinical Microbiology. 2015;**53**(10):3133-3140

[5] Murphy HM, Thomas MK, Schmidt PJ, Medeiros DT, Mcfadyen S, Pintar KDM. Estimating the burden of acute gastrointestinal illness due to *Giardia, Cryptosporidium, Campylobacter, E. coli O157* and *norovirus* associated with private wells and small water systems in Canada. Epidemiology and infection. 2016;**144**(07):1355-1370

[6] Monis PT, Caccio SM, Thompson RA. Variation in Giardia: Towards a taxonomic revision of the genus. Trends in parasitology. 2009; **25**(2): 93-100. DOI: http://dx.doi.org/10.1016/j.pt.2008.11.006

[7] Tůmová P, Uzlíková M, Wanner G, Nohýnková E. Structural organization of very small chromosomes: Study on a single-celled evolutionary distant eukaryote *Giardia intestinalis*. Chromosoma. 2015;**124**(1):81-94

[8] Pallant L, Barutzki D, Schaper R, Thompson RCA. The epidemiology of infections with Giardia species and genotypes in well cared for dogs and cats in Germany. Parasites & Vectors. 2015;**8**(1):2

[9] Thompson RCA, Ash A. Molecular epidemiology of Giardia and Cryptosporidium infections. Infection, Genetics and Evolution. 2016;**40**:315-323

[10] Birkeland SR, Preheim SP, Davids BJ, Cipriano MJ, Palm D, Reiner DS, Svärd SG, Gillin FD, McArthur AG. Transcriptome analyses of the *Giardia lamblia* life cycle. Molecular and Biochemical Parasitology. 2010;**174**(1):62-65

[11] Amorós I, Moreno Y, Reyes, Moreno-Mesonero L, Alonso JL. Prevalence of Cryptosporidium oocysts and Giardia cysts in raw and treated sewage sludges. Environmental Technology. 2016;**27**(22):2898-2904

[12] Sulemana A, Paget TA, Jarroll EL. Commitment to cyst formation in Giardia. Microbiology. **160**(2):330-339

[13] Luján HD. Giardia y giardiasis. Medicina (Buenos Aires). 2006;**66**(1):70-74

[14] Luján HD, Staffan S. Giardia: A Model Organism. Wien: Springer; 2011. 420 p

[15] Escobedo AA, Hanevik K, Almirall P, Cimerman S, Maydel A. Management of chronic *Giardia* infection. Expert Review of Anti-infective Therapy. 2014;**12**(9):1143-1157

[16] Geurden T, Vercruysse J, Claerebout E. Is Giardia a significant pathogen in production animals? Experimental Parasitology. 2010;**124**:98-106

[17] Balderrama-Carmona AP, Gortáres-Moroyoqui P, Álvarez-Valencia LH, Castro-Espinoza L, Balderas-Cortés JJ, Mondaca-Fernández I, Chaidez-Quiroz C, Meza-Montenegro MM. Quantitative microbial risk assessment of Cryptosporidium and Giardia in well water from a native community of Mexico. International Journal of Environmental Health Research. 2015;**25**(5):570-582

[18] Amorós I, Alonso JL, Cuesta G. *Cryptosporidium* oocysts and *Giardia* cysts on salad products irrigated with contaminated water. Journal of Food Protection. 2010;**73**(6):1138-1140

[19] García A, Yanko WG, Widmer G. Giardia cysts in tertiary-treated wastewater effluents: Are they infective? Water Environmental Research. 2002;**74**:541-544

[20] Caccio S, De Giacomo M, Aulicino F, Pozio E. *Giardia* cysts in wastewater treatment plants in Italy. Applied and Environmental Microbiology. 2003;**69**:3393-3398

[21] Cheng HWA, Lucy FE, Graczyk TK, Broaders MA, Tamang L, Connolly M. Fate of *Cryptosporidium parvum* and *Cryptosporidium hominis* oocysts and *Giardia duodenalis* cysts during secondary wastewater treatments. Parasitology Research. 2009;**105**:689-696. DOI: 10.1007/s00436-009-1440-y

[22] Castro-Hermida J, García-Presedo I, Almeida A, González-Warleta M, Correia Da Costa JM, Mezo M. *Cryptosporidium spp.* and *Giardia duodenalis* in two areas of Galicia (NW Spain). Science of Total Environment. 2011;**409**(13):2451-2459

[23] Donovan E, Unice K, Roberts J, Harris M, Finley B. Risk of gastrointestinal disease associated with exposure to pathogens in the water of the lower Passaic river. Applied and Environmental Microbiology. 2008;**74**:994-100

[24] Hu T. Detection of *Giardia* cysts and *Cryptosporidium* oocysts in central Taiwan Rivers by immunofluorescenceassay.JournalofMicrobiology,ImmunologyandInfection.2002;**35**(1): 68-70

[25] Ryu H, Abbaszadegan M. Long-term study of Cryptosporidium and Giardia occurrence and quantitative microbial risk assessment in surface waters of Arizona in the USA. Journal of Water Health. 2008;**06**:263-273

[26] Gortáres-Moroyoqui P, Castro-Espinoza L, Naranjo J, Karpiscak MM, Freitas RJ, Gerba CP. Microbiological water quality in a large irrigation system: El Valle del Yaqui, Sonora México. Journal of Environmental Science and Health. 2011;**46**(14):1708-1712

[27] Xiao G, Qiu Z, Qi J, Chen J, Liu F, Liu W, Liu W, Luo J, Shu W. Occurrence and potential health risk of Cryptosporidium and Giardia in the Three Gorges Reservoir, China. Water Research. 2013;**47**(7):2431-2445

[28] Karanis P, Sotiriadoua I, Kartashevc VC, Tsvetkova N, Stojanova K. Occurrence of Giardia and Cryptosporidium in water supplies of Russia and Bulgaria. Environmental Research. 2006;**102**:260-271

[29] Carmena D, Aguinagalde X, Zigorraga C, Fernández-Crespo JC, Ocio JA. Presence of Giardia cysts and Cryptosporidium oocysts in drinking water supplies in northern Spain. Journal of Applied Microbiology. 2006;**102**(3):619-629

[30] Razzolini M, Weir M, Matte M, Matte GR, Fernandes LN, Rose JB. Risk of Giardia infection for drinking water and bathing in a peri-urban area in Sao Paulo, Brazil. International Journal of Environmental Health Research. 2011;**21**(3):222-234

[31] Khaldi S, Ratajczak M, Gargala G, Fournier M, Berthe T, Favennec L, Dupont JP. Intensive exploitation of a karst aquifer leads to Cryptosporidium water supply contamination. Water Research. 2011;**45**:2906-2914

[32] Fantinatti M, Bello AM, Fernandes O, Da-Cruz AM. Identification of *Giardia lamblia* assemblage E in humans points to a new anthropozoonotic cycle. Journal of Infectious Diseases. 2016;**214**(8):1256-1259

[33] Lal A, Baker MG, Hales S, French NP. Potential effects of global environmental changes on cryptosporidiosis and giardiasis transmission. Trends in parasitology. 2013;**29**(2):83-90

[34] Adam RD. Biology of *Giardia lamblia*. Clinical Microbiology Reviews. 2001;**14**(3):447-475

[35] Alexander C, Jones B, Inverarity D, Pollock KGJ. Genotyping of *Giardia* isolates in Scotland: A descriptive epidemiological study. Epidemiology and infection. 2014;**142**(8):1636

[36] Anuar TS, Al-Mekhlafi HM, Abdul Ghani MK, Osman E, Yasin AM, Nordin A, Azreen SN, Md Salleh F, Ghazali N, Bernadus M, Moktar N. Giardiasis among different tribes of Orang Asli in Malaysia: Highlighting the presence of other family members infected with *Giardia intestinalis* as a main risk factor. International Journal for Parasitology. 2012;**42**:871-880

[37] Helmy MM, Abdel-Fattah HS, Rashed L. Real-time PCR/RFLP assay to detect *Giardia intestinalis* genotypes in human isolates with diarrhea in Egypt. Journal of Parasitology. 2009;**95**(4):1000-1004

[38] Cedillo-Rivera R, Leal YA, Yépez-Mulia L, Gómez-Delgado A, Ortega-Pierres G, Tapia-Conyer R, Muñoz O. Seroepidemiology of Giardiasis in Mexico. American Journal of Tropical Medicine and Hygiene. 2009;**80**(1):6-10

[39] Minvielle MC, Molina NB, Polverino D, Basualdo JA. First genotyping of *Giardia lamblia* from human and animal feces in Argentina, South America. Memories Institute Oswaldo Cruz, Rio de Janeiro. 2008;**103**(1):98-103

[40] Pestechian N, Rasekh H, Rostami-Nejad M, Yousofi HA, Hosseini-Safa A. Molecular identification of Giardia lamblia; is there any correlation between diarrhea and genotyping in Iranian population? Gastroenterology and Hepatology from bed to bench. 2014;**7**(3):

[41] Sprong H, Caccio SM, van der Giessen JWB. Identification of zoonotic genotypes of *Giardia duodenalis*. PLoS Neglected Tropical Disease. 2009;**3**(12):e558. DOI: 10.1371/journal.pntd.0000558

[42] Snel SJ, Baker MG, Venugopal K. The epidemiology of cryptosporidiosis in New Zealand, 1997-2006. Journal of the New Zealand Medical Association. 2009;**122**(1290):47-60

[43] Dale K, Kirk M, Sinclair M, Hall R, Leder K. Reported waterborne outbreaks of gastrointestinal disease in Australia are predominantly associated with recreational exposure in Australian and New Zealand. Journal of Public Health. 2010;**34**:527-530

[44] Daly E, Roy S, Blaney D, Manning J. Outbreak of giardiasis associated with a community drinking-water source. Epidemiology Infect. 2009;**15**:1-10

[45] Bedard BA, Elder R, Phillips L, Wachunas MF. Giardia outbreak associated with a roadside spring in Rensselaer County, New York. Epidemiology and Infection. 2016;**144**(14):3013-3016

[46] Karon A, Hanni K, Mohle-Boetani J, Beretti R, Hill V, Arrowood M, Johnston S, Xiao L, Vugia D. Giardiasis outbreak at a camp after installation of a slow-sand filtration system. Epidemiology Infection. 2010;**29**:1-5

[47] Tuncay S, Delibas S, Inceboz T, Over L, Oral AM, Akisu C, Aksoy U. An outbreak of gastroenteritis associated with intestinal parasites. Turkey Society of Parasitology. 2008;**32**:249-252

[48] Nygard K, Schimmer B, Sobstad O, Walde A, Tveit I, Langeland N, Hausken T, Aavitsland P. A large community outbreak of waterborne giardiasis-delayed detection in a non-endemic urban area. BMC Public Health. 2006;**6**:141

[49] Yoder JS, Beach MJ. *Cryptosporidiosis* Surveillance—United States, 2003-2005 and *Giardiasis* Surveillance—United States, 2003-2005, In Morbidity and Mortality Weekly Report 2, 56 (SS-7). CDC, Atlanta, GA, US: Editorial Board; 2007

[50] Logue C, Barbieri NL, Nielsen DW. Pathogens of food animals: Sources, characteristics, human risk, and methods of detection. Advances in Food and Nutrition Research. 2017. DOI: 10.1016/bs.afnr.2016.12.009

[51] Schijven J, de Roda A. A survey of diving behavior and accidental water ingestion among Dutch occupational and sport divers to assess the risk of infection with waterborne pathogenic microorganisms. Environmental Health Perspectives. 2006;**1**:712-717

[52] Utaaker KS, Huang Q, Robertson LJ. A reduced-cost approach for analyzing fresh produce for contamination with *Cryptosporidium* oocysts and/or *Giardia* cysts. Food Research International. 2015;**77**:326-332

[53] Fundora HH, Puig PY, Chiroles RS, Rodríguez BAM, Gallardo DJ, Milián SY. Métodos inmunológicos utilizados en la identificación rápida de bacterias y protozoarios en aguas. Revista Cubana de Higiene y Epidemiología. 2013;**51**(1):84-96

[54] United States Environmental Protection Agency (USEPA). ICR Microbial laboratory Manual. ICR Protozoan Method for Detecting *Giardi*a Cyst and *Cryptosporidium* Oocyst. Cincinnati, OH: USEPA; 1996

[55] de Oliveira Pinto D, Urbano L, Neto RC. Immunomagnetic separation study applied to detection of Giardia spp. cysts and Cryptosporidium spp. oocysts in water samples. Water Science and Technology: Water Supply. 2016;**16**(1):144-149

[56] Singhal S, Mittal V, Khare V, Singh YI. Comparative analysis of enzyme-linked immunosorbent assay and direct microscopy for the diagnosis of *Giardia intestinalis* in fecal samples. Indian Journal of Pathology and Microbiology. 2015;**58**(1):69

[57] Dyab AK, Yones DA, Sayed DM, Hassan TM. Detection, enumeration and viability evaluation of *Giardia* cysts in water samples using flow. Cytometry. 2015;**4**(6):077-086

[58] Weir MH, Mitchell J, Flynn W, Pope JM. Development of a microbial dose response visualization and modelling application for QMRA modelers and educators. Environmental Modelling and Software. 2017;**88**:74-83

[59] Romero-Barrios P, Hempen M, Messens W, Stella P, Hugas M. Quantitative microbiological risk assessment (QMRA) of food-borne zoonoses at the European level. Food Control. 2013;**29**(2):343-349

[60] Hunter PR, Anderle de Sylor M, Risebro HL, Gordon LN, Kay D, Hartemann P. Quantitative microbial risk assessment of Cryptosporidiosis and Giardiasis from very small private water supplies. Risk Analysis. 2011;**31**(2):228-236

[61] USEPA. Surface Water Treatment Rules [Internet]. 1989 [Updated: 2016]. Available from: www.epa.gov [Accessed: 2017]

[62] VROM. Waterleidingbesluit (Drinking water decree), Ministery of Housing. The Hague, The Netherlands: Physical Planning and the Environment; 2001

[63] Schets FM, van Wijnen JH, Schijven JF, Schoon H, de Roda AMH. Monitoring of waterborne pathogens in surface waters in Amsterdam, The Netherlands, and the potential health risk associated with exposure to *Cryptosporidium* and *Giardia* in these waters. Applied and Environmental Microbiology. 2008;**74**(7):2069-2078

[64] Carlander A, Schonning C, Stenstrom TA. Energy forest irrigated with wastewater: A comparative microbial risk assessment. Journal of Water and Health. 2009;**07**(3):413-433

[65] Mota A, Mena KD, Soto-Beltran M, Tarwater P, Chaidez C. Risk assessment of Cryptosporidium and Giardia in water irrigation fresh produce in Mexico. Journal of Food Protection. 2009;**72**(10):2184-2188

[66] Soller J, Bartrand T, Ashbolt N, Ravenscroft J, Wade TJ. Estimating the primary etiologic agents in recreational freshwaters impacted by human sources of faecal contamination. Water Research. 2010;**44**(16):4736-4747

[67] Ahmed W, Vieritz A, Goonetilleke A, Gardner T. Health risk from the use of roof-harvested rainwater in Southeast Queensland, Australia, as potable or nonpotable water, determined using quantitative microbial risk assessment. Applied and Environmental Microbiology. 2010;**76**(22):7382-7391

[68] Sato MIZ, Galvani AT, Padula JA, Nardocci AC, de Souza Lauretto M, Razzolini MTP, Hachich EM. Assessing the infection risk of *Giardia* and *Cryptosporidium* in public drinking water delivered by surface water systems in Sao Paulo State, Brazil. Science of Total Environment. 2013;**442**:389-396

[69] Betancourt W, Duarte D, Vásquez R, Gurian P. *Cryptosporidium* and *Giardia* in tropical recreational marine waters contaminated with domestic sewage: Estimation of bathing-associated disease risks. Marine Pollution Bulletin. 2014;**85**(1):268-273

[70] Yapo R, Koné B, Bonfoh B, Cissé G, Zinsstag J, Nguyen-Viet H. Quantitative microbial risk assessment related to urban wastewater and lagoon water reuse in Abidjan, Côte d'Ivoire. Journal of Water and Health. 2014;**12**(2):301-309

[71] USEPA. Exposure Factors Handbook. Washington, DC, National Center for Environmental Assessment, Office of Research and Development; 1997 (EPA/600/P-95/002Fa,b,c)

[72] Haas CN, Rose JB, Gerba CP. Quantitative Microbial Risk Assessment. 1st ed. New York: John Wiley & Sons, Inc.; 1999

[73] Barbeau B, Payment P, Coallier J, Clement B, Prevost M. Evaluating the risk of infection from the presence of *Giardia* and *Cryptosporidium* in drinking water. Quantitative Microbiology. 2000;**2**:37-54

[74] Ryu H, Alum A, Mena KD, Abbaszadegan M. Assessment of the risk of infection by *Cryptosporidium* and *Giardia* in non-potable reclaimed water. Water Science Technology. 2007;**55**(1-2):283-290

[75] Sterk G, ten Veldhuis JAE, Clemens FLHR, Berends BR. Microbial risk assessment for urban pluvial flooding, In: 11th International Conference on Urban Drainage, Edinburgh, Scotland, UK, 2008

[76] An W, Zhang D, Xiao S, Yu J, Yang M. Risk assessment of Giardia in rivers of southern China based on continuous monitoring. Journal of Environmental Science. 2012;**24**(2):309-313

[77] Zhang Y, Chen Z, An W, Xiao S, Yuan H, Zhang D, Yang M. Risk assessment of *Giardia* from a full scale MBR sewage treatment plant caused by membrane integrity failure. Journal of Environmental Sciences. 2015;**30**:252-258

[78] Sheludchenko M, Padovan A, Katouli M, Stratton H. Removal of Fecal Indicators, Pathogenic Bacteria, *Adenovirus*, *Cryptosporidium* and *Giardia* (oo)cysts in Waste Stabilization Ponds in Northern and Eastern Australia. International Journal of Environmental Research and Public Health. 2016;**13**:96. DOI: 10.3390/ijerph13010096

[79] Nasser AM, Huberman Z, Zilberman A, Greenfeld S. Die-off and retardation of *Cryptosporidium* spp. oocyst in loamy soil saturated with secondary effluent. Water Science and Technology. Water Supply. 2003;**3**(4):253-259

[80] Unuabonah EI, Taubert A. Clay–polymer nanocomposites (CPNs): Adsorbents of the future for water treatment. Applied Clay Science. 2014. DOI: 10.1016/j.clay.2014.06.016

[81] Bondi M, Messi P, Prakash MH, Papadopoulou C, Niederhausern S. Emerging microbial concerns in food safety and new control measures. BioMed Research International. 2014. DOI: 10.1155/2014/251512

[82] United States Department of Agriculture/Food Safety and Inspection Service (USDA/FSIS) and USEPA. Microbial Risk Assessment Guideline: Pathogenic Organisms with Focus on Food and Water. 2012FSIS Publication No. USDA/FSIS/2012-001; EPA Publication No. EPA/100/J12/001

[83] Escobedo AA, Almirall P, Rumbaute R, Rodríguez-Morales AJ. Potential impact of macroclimatic variability on the epidemiology of giardiasis in three provinces of Cuba, 2010-2012. Journal of Infection and Public Health. 2015;**8**:80-89. DOI: 10.1016/j.jiph.2014.06.001

[84] Wu X, Lu Y, Zhou S, Chen L, Xu B. Impact of climate change on human infectious diseases: Empirical evidence and human adaptation. Environmental International. 2016;**86**:14-23